Eat To Beat…
ACNE!

How a plant-based diet can help heal your skin.

Leigh Matthews BA Hons, NT Dip. HE.

Contents

Chapter 1:   Getting to know your skin.

Chapter 2:   How to avoid common causes of acne.

Chapter 3:   Is there any truth to these skin myths?

Chapter 4:   Got milk? Got acne?

Chapter 5:   Do cleanses really work for spot-prone skin?

Chapter 6:   Inflammation and acne.

Chapter 7:   Anti-inflammatory foods.

Chapter 8:   More skin-solutions - from your pantry!

Preface

Fasting, purging, dieting, cleansing, detoxing - all buzzwords designed to draw you in with the promise of revolutionising your health and your life with little effort required on your part. Sadly, these fads and miracle products promise more than they can really provide. In fact, some quick fixes can irritate your skin and leave your overall health in much poorer shape than before.

Why is this the case? Well, when it comes to health, especially skin health, extreme food fads and health trends can disrupt the normal functioning of your body, leading to irritation, inflammation, and a decreased ability to heal and repair damaged skin.

A 10-day juice fast, clear soup cleanse, or Master Cleanse encourage the idea that years of unhealthy living can be counteracted simply by following one extreme dietary plan for a few days. The truth is that these cleanses often place extreme stress on the body, are decidedly unhealthy, and typically act only as a salve to someone's conscience before they slip back into old unhealthy habits.

The real way to achieve and maintain good health is to establish and maintain healthy habits. Indeed, it is unlikely that anything other than simple healthy eating will clear up your acne and improve your general health.

The problem we have then is how we define 'simple healthy eating', and how to go about sticking to such a diet, not as a fad but as a way of life. Not only does the science support a plant-based diet as the healthier option for long-term health, there are numerous other benefits to such a diet that can offer added motivation to persevere even when old habits appear tempting.

Some of the positive changes associated with eating a plant-based diet can happen quickly, while others can take a little longer to become noticeable. For example, switching to a plant-based diet can help improve sluggish digestion, decrease inflammation, and help with blood sugar regulation, resulting in more stable energy levels. Over time, a healthy plant-based diet typically leads to better blood lipid status (including cholesterol levels), improved blood pressure, and the achievement and maintenance of a healthy body weight and Body Mass Index, whatever that looks like for you.

The important thing is to recognise that the skin is just one of the body's organs, albeit the largest, and so what affects your overall health also affects your skin. While a healthy, plant-based diet doesn't promise an acne cure overnight, the advantage of this approach is that positive changes are sustainable because they also support better overall health and well-being. Other treatments for acne may help clear up the skin in the short-term, but at the expense of overall health, making such interventions inherently difficult to maintain and highly questionable.

By making some basic changes in your food philosophy (and in your pantry) you can save time and money, feel less overwhelmed by stress, sleep better, and see your skin begin to radiate with good health. And, as you'll already be investing in the best detox strategy of all, namely your liver, you'll have all the motivation you need to avoid jumping on the next so-called miracle diet.

In the following chapters we will examine some common myths connecting skin and diet; why your skin needs more than just a three day cleanse every now and then; and how fasting and detoxing could actually harm your skin and trigger acne breakouts. We'll start by getting to know our skin, and we'll finish with a look at how to create simple products for on-the-spot acne relief using basic pantry items.

This book will provide you with the tools you need to choose skin-healthy foods every day – essentially, you'll learn how to eat to beat acne!

CHAPTER ONE: GETTING TO KNOW YOUR SKIN.

Chances are that you're reading this book because you're struggling with acne. Maybe you get the occasional flare-up and are looking for ways to keep things under control, or it could be that severe acne has caused your self-confidence to plummet and is ruining your quality of life. Acne is a major issue for many teens and young adults, and while adolescent acne typically clears up in the early twenties, an estimated 14% of women aged 25 to 50 continue to suffer from acne (Balta et al., 2013). Even those whose teenage acne clears up may experience a recurrence of the skin condition in the premenopausal period when hormone levels begin to fluctuate once again.

Where acne persists into adulthood and/or is severe it is often an outward indication of ongoing hormonal dysfunction, nutrient deficiency, chronic systemic inflammation, immune system irregularities, metabolic disorders, or even high levels of immunoglobulin factor-1 (IGF-1), a substance associated with a range of health issues and which dramatically increases your risk of cancer (Melnik & Schmitz, 2009).

Taking care of your skin is not, therefore, a matter of simple vanity or indulgence. Skin health is almost always an indication of general health and can act as an early warning sign for serious underlying health issues. What's on the outside might not matter much in terms of the content of your character but it could be an important prompt to improve a number of markers for good health. The added bonus is, of course, that improving overall health can lead to you looking and feeling great.

Embarking on any successful health journey requires a little preliminary research, time to strategise, and a good deal of motivation. Before you jump ahead to the sections of this book that show you which plant foods offer the greatest benefits for skin health, it's important to know a little about how your skin actually works.

What Your Skin Does for You

The skin is the largest organ in the body, weighing as much as a small dog (around 5 kg or 11 lbs) and measuring around two square metres (22 square feet) in adults. The trouble is that we often take our skin for granted until problems arise, despite our skin performing a huge number of tasks that help keep us healthy inside and out. These important functions of the skin include:

- Regulating body temperature and hydration
- Protecting against infection
- Producing melanin to absorb damaging ultraviolet radiation
- Eliminating excess oils, toxins and other substances
- Producing vitamin D
- Alerting us to painful stimuli

Our skin also helps us communicate (whether we like it or not), and can reflect our inner emotional state through blushing, turning pale, and sweating.

The health of the skin is influenced by what you eat and drink, the medications you take, the shampoos, body lotions, soaps and cosmetics you use, and even the clothing you wear and the furniture you sit and sleep on. The appearance and health of your skin is also at the mercy of environmental factors such as air pollution, humidity, sun exposure, wind, and daily knocks and scrapes. Understanding how the skin functions and how it can reflect what is happening on the inside of the body means that you will never look at spots, wrinkles, dry skin, psoriasis, or rosacea in quite the same way again.

The Skin as Sentinel

Many internal diseases and conditions have an effect on the skin, and dermatologists are often the first to note the possibility of gastrointestinal distress, an autoimmune condition, hormonal imbalance, or other abnormality.

Nutritionists, dietitians, and naturopaths will typically take a good long look at their patients' skin to help guide their diagnoses and monitor the effects of treatments, even when they are not directly addressing skin issues. This is because good habits for naturally healthy skin are usually good habits for general health. Learning the secret language of your skin can offer early warning signs of infection, disease or distress.

The Structure of the Skin

The skin is a complex organ that has to contend with a variety of insults from both the external environment and the interior workings of the body. The skin's surface is covered in dead skin cells that continually slough off to reveal new skin cells below. The uppermost layer of living skin cells is called the epidermis ('epi' meaning on or over in Latin and 'dermis' meaning skin). Beneath the epidermis is the dermis itself, which is mainly made up of collagen and elastin. The dermis contains blood vessels, nerve endings, sebaceous glands, and sweat glands.

Acne often arises due to blockages of the sebaceous glands caused by an accumulation of dead or damaged skin cells. This may be an indication of an underlying problem of hyperplasia (where the skin cells divide and grow abnormally fast), or it may a localised reaction to bacterial invasion. Underneath the dermis is a layer of adipose tissue (fat), which cushions the internal organs and bones.

The Epidermis
The Horny Layer

There are four layers within the epidermis, the uppermost being the stratum corneum, or 'horny layer'. The reason for this moniker is that the cells of the stratum corneum primarily contain keratin, a strong protein produced by keratinocytes and also found in the nails and the hair. The cells of the stratum corneum also include lipids (fats) that help the skin to retain moisture and regulate the passage of substances in and out of the body.

The stratum corneum is thinner than a human hair but these cells are exceptionally tough and form an integral part of the body's barrier to the outside world. The cells forming the stratum corneum flake off or are exfoliated during everyday activities, and are constantly being replaced. New cells form in the deeper basal layer of the epidermis and migrate upwards to the outermost layer.

In most people, the epidermis is completely renewed every six to ten weeks but those with psoriasis may have a process that takes as little as four days. This rapid cell turnover leads to an excess of stratum corneum cells and is what causes the scaly appearance characteristic of psoriasis. Rapid cell turnover in the skin can also lead to blocked pores and inflammation, resulting in acne-like lesions.

The Granular Layer

The stratum granulosum lies directly beneath the stratum corneum, with the exception of the skin on our palms and soles of our feet where an extra layer, the stratum lucidum, separates the stratum granulosum and stratum corneum.

The granular layer also contains keratinocytes that produce keratin, but these keratinocytes have lost their nuclei (the brain of the cell), and are in their final stage of life. As these cells break down they release their contents into the extracellular space between the cells. The contents, or cytoplasm, of the cells in this layer of the skin has a granular (grain-like) appearance, hence its name as the stratum granulosum.

Inside the keratinocytes are organelles called lamellar bodies that release lipids to be used in the creation of a lipid barrier or cell membrane. The lipid cell membrane is formed by an arrangement of polar and non-polar lipids parallel to the cell surface. The arrangement and type of lipids (fats) in these cell membranes has a huge effect on the health of the cells. This is just one of the reasons why a diet full of saturated fats (typically found in animal products) can adversely affect the skin.

Monounsaturated and polyunsaturated fats from plant-foods are essential for keeping skin cell membranes flexible and functional. These healthy fats also support the cell membranes in their responsibility to facilitate proper communication between cells. Healthy cell membranes are also better able to control what goes in and out of the cells. This means that cells with functional membranes are less likely to allow toxins to enter the cells, and are better able to eject toxins, as well as being quicker at taking up much-needed nutrients to fuel important cellular processes.

The Spinous Layer

The stratum spinosum is the layer of the epidermis below the stratum granulosum. In this layer, the keratinocytes begin to produce the aforementioned lamellar bodies, which are enriched with polar lipids, glycophospholipids, free sterols, phospholipids and catabolic enzymes. As we just saw, these lamellar bodies release their lipids once they migrate up into the granular layer.

The keratinocytes in the stratum spinosum are connected through desmosomes, specialised cell structures that aid cell-to-cell adhesion and which prevent the cells shearing. Genetic mutations that affect desmosome function can result in skin conditions such as Darier's disease and Hopf's disease. Abnormalities of desmosome function can also lead to cardiac problems as desmosomes are also essential for helping cells stick together throughout the body.

Langerhans cells can be found in the middle of the stratum spinosum and these cells form part of the immune system. Langerhans cells take in foreign bodies (such as bacteria) and present them to other cells of the immune system, such as monocytes, in order to prompt an immune system response and production of antibodies against infection. When the cells are unable to quickly eliminate toxic metabolites, or are starved of adequate nutrition, healthy circulation, or oxygen, Langerhans cells may become dysfunctional. This means that the Langerhans cells might respond abnormally to the body's own cells, triggering autoimmune skin diseases such as scleroderma.

The Basal Layer

The lowest layer of the epidermis is the basal layer, also known as the germinal layer or stratum germinativum. This layer of the skin is mostly made up of proliferating and non-proliferating keratinocytes. These keratin-producing cells are attached to the basement membrane that separates the epidermis from the dermis by hemidesmosomes.

Melanocytes are also found in the stratum basale. These are the cells that produce melanin, the pigment responsible for the colour of our skin. One skin complaint, commonly known as blackheads, is a result of the skin's pores becoming blocked with melanin, illustrating how the health of even the deepest layers of the epidermis can affect the skin's outward appearance. Melanocytes are connected to other layers of the epidermis through dendrites (long nerve cells).

Merkel cells (another type of nerve cell) are also found in this layer of the skin, and are especially abundant in our fingertips and lips where they are involved in the sensation of light touch.

A basement membrane separates the epidermis from the dermis, and this type of membrane also lines the cavities containing our organs, as well as the endothelium that lines the inside of our blood vessels.

The Dermis

Despite its four layers (or five layers - in the palms and soles), the epidermis is actually relatively thin compared to the dermis, which makes up the majority of the skin. Within the dermis are blood vessels, connective tissues, lymph vessels, elastin and collagen fibres, and living skin cells. Nerve cells, hair follicles, sebaceous glands, and sweat glands are also present in the dermis, with pores opening out onto the skin's surface to control secretions.

Sebaceous Glands

With the exception of the palms, soles and tops of the feet, sebaceous glands are found all over the body, varying in size depending on their location. Sebaceous glands on the face and chest are bigger, for example, than those on the arms and legs, but they all open out into hair follicles or directly onto the skin. The purpose of the sebaceous glands is to produce sebum, an oily substance that lubricates the hair and keeps the skin hydrated by preventing excessive water-loss.

Although sebum helps keep the skin clear of some kinds of bacteria, it is also implicated in the build-up of some bacteria. The rate of sebum production is hormone-dependent, which is one reason why the hormonal upheaval experienced in puberty can lead to acne. In such cases, sebum may clog pores and promote infection, causing the angry red pustules associated with back acne and acne in the T-zone formed by the brow, nose, and chin. This is also why hormone dysregulation that continues into, or begins, in adulthood can result in chronic adult acne. Such hormone disruption is often linked to diet and lifestyle.

Sweat Glands and Lymph Nodes

The dermis is also the site of the sweat glands and lymph vessels, along with fibroblasts, melanocytes, and other types of cells. An average human body has around four million sweat glands which are responsible for regulating body temperature and helping eliminate some toxins and metabolic waste. Dehydration can have a profound effect on the ability of the skin to eliminate toxins efficiently, leading to a build-up of unwanted waste in the dermis.

The number of sweat glands varies between sites on the body with an abundance of such glands on the palms and soles. Homeostatic mechanisms respond to an increase in body temperature by opening up sweat glands onto the pores of the skin in order to secrete water and other substances. As the water on the skin evaporates, the skin begins to cool, prompting the closure of the pores in order to maintain body temperature. This ongoing cycle of pores opening and closing is essential for effective regulation of optimal body temperature.

The Lymphatic System

Lymph vessels do not excrete substances out onto the skin but, instead, drain excess fluid between cells and deal with threats to the body, such as bacteria or viruses. Unlike the circulatory system that pumps blood around the body, lymphatic drainage relies on the regular contraction and relaxation of muscles during daily activities to squeeze and push lymphatic fluid through the vast network of lymph vessels and nodes. The lymphatic system also transports fats and fat-soluble nutrients including vitamins A, D, E, K, and B12, and carotenoids such as beta-carotene around the body after they are absorbed in the gut.

What is Lymph and why do Lymph Nodes Swell?

Lymph fluid is a mix of white blood cells, fats, water, and proteins. Dehydration, excess dietary fat (particularly saturated fat, found in abundance in animal products), and inadequate protein can all contribute to a sluggish lymphatic drainage system. This results in poorer immune system function, swollen lymph nodes, and skin issues, such as acne, from toxic build-up.

When an organism such as a virus or bacteria attack the body, our immune system works to trap the invader in the lymph nodes. This is so that our immune system cells can concentrate their attack and more effectively fight off the potential infection. This accumulation of immune system cells and bacteria results in enlargement of the lymph nodes during an infection, and as the infection is dealt with the dead bacteria or other organisms are flushed through the lymphatic system and eliminated from the body.

Lymph nodes remain swollen for a little while after infection as it takes time for the concentration of white blood cells and other immune system components to dissipate. When lymph nodes are repeatedly enlarged this can be a sign of persistent or repeated infection, or may indicate a problem with the immune system, possibly due to impaired zinc status or a deficiency of some other nutrient(s). Poor skin hygiene may also be a factor, along with sluggish lymphatic drainage, offering ample opportunities for improving skin health through diet and external skin care.

Figuring Out Your Acne Flare-Ups

As you can see, the skin is a complex organ, meaning that it is almost impossible to fully understand how your daily choices and interactions will affect the health of your skin. This does not mean, however, that it is a pointless endeavour to try to make the best choices you can, given the current state of medical knowledge.

It is all too easy to get caught up in living day-to-day and then be caught off guard by poor skin health, or poor general health. When this happens it is tempting to throw blame at one potential culprit and ignore everything else that is playing a role in sabotaging health and happiness.

The trick, then, is to learn to practice mindfulness, figure out what may have gone awry, and develop healthy habits to address the overall picture. Of course, acne and other skin complaints can be an indication of a more serious underlying issue that requires professional intervention, and it is important to know when to seek medical assistance. In many cases though, you can dramatically improve your skin health by taking a little time to sit back and reassess how you're living, and what you're putting on and in your body on a daily basis.

You can probably recall a time when you felt overwhelmed by a series of rapid life changes that then led to a period of ill health, or suboptimal health. Perhaps you were in the process of moving house when an exciting job opportunity arose that you couldn't pass up. With so much to do, maybe you set your alarm a little early, had an extra cup of coffee mid-morning, and then had another little pick-me-up when tiredness hit around 3pm. Perhaps you added a pastry to that coffee break, just to get you through to the end of work, at which point you realise you don't have the energy to make dinner, so you head out for dinner with friends instead and have a couple of drinks to unwind. When you wake up at 2am, feeling thirsty and exhausted, it's a challenge to get back to sleep as you're already thinking about the next day. Unable to turn off your racing mind, you sleep fitfully for a few more hours until your alarm sounds and you wake up exhausted and desperate for coffee. After a few weeks of this, with new job stress and new people to socialise with, you don't even realise that you're now drinking several cups of coffee a day, eating lots of simple carbohydrates because you need quick energy, and have upped your alcohol intake to help you sleep and unwind.

If this sounds at all familiar, and your skin health is suffering, it may be time to invest in working out what needs to change in your life to get you back on track and feeling healthy and energised. Perhaps you have been tempted to try to conceal your acne with make-up, or maybe you have been throwing money at your skin by way of expensive face creams, lotions, and cleansers. These approaches may help a little but they fail to address the underlying cause(s) of acne, and the success of these 'cures' is likely to be short-lived, if they work at all.

Whether you like it or not, you are in a relationship for life with your skin, and the key to any healthy relationship is communication. So, look over the questions on the following page and give yourself some time to ask what it is that your skin is trying to tell you.

Practical Steps

Whenever you have a skin breakout, it can help to ask yourself:

1. Am I under more stress than usual?
2. Has my diet changed in the past few days, weeks, or months?
3. Am I drinking more alcohol, coffee, or sugary drinks than usual?
4. How's my digestion?
5. How much and how well am I sleeping?
6. Have I changed my shampoo, soap, moisturiser, or other toiletries?
7. Is my make-up old and likely to be harbouring bacteria?
8. Am I drinking enough water?
9. Have I started a new job, moved house, or started a new hobby/sport?
10. How's my general health? Am I easily tired, in pain, feeling grumpy and depressed?

Oftentimes, the culprit for skin flare-ups can be found by working through this checklist, especially when your skin health is usually pretty good but has taken a bit of a hit recently. It really could be as simple as the fact that you ran out of your usual soap, started using something else that dries out your skin, and now have dehydrated skin that is vulnerable to cracking and subsequent infection. Or, maybe you became hooked on a new TV show and missed out on some sleep, meaning that your skin, and the rest of your body, just hasn't had sufficient downtime in which to repair and heal.

Work through these questions and see if there is a likely culprit, then make a realistic plan to tackle the issue. This may mean a simple change, such as taking a bottle of water to work and drinking the whole thing by the end of your day. Or, it could be more involved, necessitating an appointment with a therapist or physician to get support in making changes to drinking habits, or how you handle stress. Keep a symptom diary for acne flare-ups, and a brief daily journal to track progress – you might be surprised what correlations show up.

CHAPTER TWO: HOW TO AVOID COMMON CAUSES OF ACNE.

Now you've read chapter one and become a little better acquainted with your skin, you're in a good position to begin spotting tell-tale signs of underlying health issues. Spotting these signs will quickly become second nature, allowing you to anticipate and better prevent skin issues arising, or simply giving you the information you need to quickly address a problem if a pimple does poke its way through.

Let's take a look at the three main causative factors of acne:

1. Increased levels of circulating androgens (sex hormones)
2. Follicular hyperkeratinisation (rapid skin cell turnover) leading to blocked sebum glands
3. Bacterial skin infection (with Propionibacterium acnes) leading to localised inflammation.

It should be pretty clear from this list that we cannot simply say that eating chocolate causes acne, and to cure acne we just need to cut out chocolate. In a roundabout way, eating chocolate can contribute to acne flare-ups, as we'll see in the next chapter, because someone who eats lots of sugar-laden dairy milk chocolate will typically experience blood sugar spikes and increased inflammation that negatively impact skin health. This isn't, however, the whole picture, with acne pathogenesis usually a little more nuanced than blaming a candy bar.

By examining the underlying factors that can lead to follicular hyperkeratinisation and increased levels of circulating androgens (including testosterone), we soon run up against a possible culprit worthy of exploration, namely metabolic syndrome.

What is Metabolic Syndrome?

Metabolic syndrome refers to a group of conditions and diseases that share an underlying contributing factor, the dysregulation of insulin and glucose metabolism. For a long time conditions include atherosclerosis, coronary artery disease, type 2 diabetes, and hypertension were considered isolated issues, but now these, and acne vulgaris, can be counted amongst the symptoms of metabolic syndrome. This is because these health problems are associated with fundamental functional imbalances of blood sugar from excessive consumption of refined foods and a sedentary lifestyle leading to systemic inflammation, insulin resistance, and problems of glycation.

If you think back to the example given at the end of chapter one, you'll recall that managing stress and pressure by drinking coffee and eating sweet, sugary snacks can lead to erratic energy levels and cravings for more simple carbohydrates and caffeine. Excessive intake of carbohydrate results in blood sugar spikes that the body will try to manage by releasing large amounts of insulin. Insulin is a hormone that directs glucose (sugar) out of the blood and into cells, including muscle cells as stored energy. This helps to keep blood glucose levels low and reduce the likelihood of damage caused by undesirable glycation of proteins.

However, when insulin production is triggered over and over again by excess dietary carbohydrate consumption this can cause our cells to stop responding properly to the hormone. Known as insulin resistance, this lack of response means that the cells no longer take up glucose from the blood, leaving the cells starved of fuel, and blood sugar persistently elevated.

When muscle cells have problems taking up glucose this can lead to early onset of fatigue. A few subpar gym performances, a lack of energy, and increasing fat stores can all indicate a problem with insulin sensitivity.

In response to this plummet in efficient energy production, the body may trigger carbohydrate cravings and release yet more insulin, flooding the system and compounding the problem. In order to escape from this vicious downward spiral into metabolic syndrome, steps need to be taken to reverse insulin resistance and ensure that the fuel we're taking in is used properly to produce energy.

A range of other processes are also involved in blood sugar management. These processes can, for a while at least, help control blood glucose levels and maintain a certain level of function and energy. Eventually, however, repeated exposure to these spikes in blood sugar can cause insulin-producing cells (pancreatic beta cells) to burn out, leaving the body unable to respond properly to control blood sugar. This is when blood glucose levels can begin to rise dramatically, leading to the manifestation of type 2 diabetes.

A Low GI Diet for Acne

What does all this have to do with acne? Well, in a recent study involving 248 participants aged 18-25, people with moderate to severe acne had higher dietary GI (Glycaemic Index), more added sugar, and higher levels of total sugar, than people with mild acne or no acne at all (Burris et al., 2014). This group also consumed more servings of milk per day, more saturated fat, and more trans-fat, but only 58% of the study's participants thought that their diet influenced their acne.

What this study suggests is that it may be possible to get control of your acne by improving your understanding of how dietary and lifestyle choices influence the development of metabolic syndrome. By working on effective strategies to combat or prevent metabolic syndrome, you could begin to address many of the factors involved in poor skin health, such as inflammation and hormone dysregulation.

To reduce insulin resistance it is recommended to eat unrefined sources of carbohydrate that are digested more slowly, so as to release a steady amount of manageable glucose. This helps avoid overtaxing the body's blood sugar homeostatic controls, i.e. a slower release of carbohydrate from food means that less insulin is needed overall. This then means that the body's cells are less likely to become resistant to the chemical messenger through overexposure to insulin.

Combining lower GI foods with protein and fat looks like the best approach for reducing hyperinsulinaemia, insulin resistance, and metabolic syndrome. This is because the combination of tehse macronutrients helps to slow down digestion and thereby support healthy blood sugar regulation. This type of diet works best when dietary carbohydrates are not refined and when fibre content is high.

In one analysis of 11 medium to long-term studies using the glycemic index (GI) approach to diabetes and lipid management, all but one study noted benefits from a low GI diet (Brand-Miller, 1994). Low GI diets led to average reductions of 16% for day-long blood glucose, 9% for glycosylated hemoglobin, 6% for cholesterol, and 9% for triglycerides, showing that diet can improve a range of measures in regards to metabolic syndrome.

If you're not familiar with the glycaemic index, this is simply a way of measuring the rate at which foods lead to increases in blood sugar. Basic glucose has a glycaemic index score of 100 and provides the standard against which other foods can be compared. For example, the GI of pumpernickel bread is around 51, while the GI of a plain white baguette is around 95. In general, the more fibre, good fats, and proteins a food contains the lower its GI, making whole foods the best option for maintaining consistent blood sugar levels.

The average vegetarian or vegan has a higher carbohydrate intake than the average omnivore, but vegetarians and vegans usually also have a lower incidence of insulin resistance. At first glance, this might not make much sense, but the reality is that the majority of people eating a plant-based diet have a high intake of low GI sources of carbohydrate, such as vegetables and whole grains.

In a single-blinded, parallel intervention study, teens and young-adults with acne had dramatically decreased acne scores after eating a low GI diet for just 12 weeks (Smith et al., 2007). The trial involved 43 men aged 15-25 who followed a low-glycemic-load diet composed of 25% energy from protein and 45% from low-glycemic-index carbohydrates, while the controls ate a diet that emphasised carbohydrate-dense foods without any mention of the glycemic index. Acne lesion counts decreased by 23.5 in the low GI group, compared to a reduction of just 12 in the control group. Insulin sensitivity also improved in the low GI group, offering further advantages for skin health and general well-being. The low GI diet also led to an average 2.9 kg reduction in body weight and a 0.92 decrease in Body Mass Index (BMI) compared to 0.5 kg, and 0.01 BMI, respectively, in the control group.

As we mentioned a moment ago, insulin doesn't act in isolation. Instead, blood sugar control and insulin levels are closely associated with the production, secretion, and function of other hormones such as testosterone, oestrogen, and growth hormone. A high level of circulating insulin also affects the synthesis of immunoglobulin-factor binding protein-1 (IGFBP-1) which leads to an increased level of IGF-1 itself. IGF-1 increases the synthesis of protein in the cells, triggers cellular hypertrophy (excessively large cell growth), inhibits the normal process of clearing away damaged cells through cell death (apoptosis), and increases cell proliferation (the rate at which cells divide). As such,

IGF-1 is linked to the development and progression of cancer, and is also associated with skin conditions that result from rapid cell growth (Arnaldez & Helman, 2012). Some studies have concluded that a vegan diet can help counteract this increased cancer risk by lowering IGF-1 levels (McCarty, 1999).

In summary, a high GI diet, full of refined carbohydrates such as sugar or white flour, can promote acne by way of high insulin levels, increased IGF-1, and the resulting effect of rapidly growing skin cells that don't know when to die and slough off. In such a situation, pores can become clogged with dead or damaged cells and sebum, paving the way for bacterial infection, inflammation, and pus-filled pimples and blackheads.

Insulin, Androgens, and Acne

Now we know all about how metabolic syndrome can lead to blackheads, let's back up for a second and take a look at the list at the beginning of the chapter. The first item on the list is high circulating levels of androgens. What does this mean and how is it connected to insulin and diet?

Firstly, hyperinsulinaemia (consistently elevated insulin levels) resulting from repeated excessive consumption of high GI foods decreases the production of IGFBP-1. This leads to increasing tissue levels of IGF-1, which then stimulates androgen synthesis in the ovaries and testes. IGF-1 can simultaneously reduce the production of sex hormone binding globulin (SHBG) in the liver, leading to high levels of circulating sex hormones which directly contribute to acne vulgaris (Bebakar et al., 1990).

Specifically, low levels of SHBG are associated with an increased ratio of testosterone to oestrogen and, subsequently, to hirsutism (excess hair growth), polycystic ovary syndrome (PCOS), and acne vulgaris (Hays, 2005).

SHBG synthesis is also decreased simply by excess sugar in the diet, rather than just through elevated insulin. This is because sugar can be converted to fat in the liver through a process that also reduces blood SHBG levels.

In addition to the interaction between diet and SHBG, researchers at Harvard recently explored an apparent connection between endometriosis and acne. These scientists found that women with a history of severe teenage acne were 20% more likely than their peers to develop endometriosis (Xie, et al., 2014). The researchers recommended that anyone with a history of severe teenage acne who also had irregular menstruation or abdominal pain should be evaluated for endometriosis, a condition which affects approximately one in ten women but which is typically only diagnosed several years after onset. As acne is an easily observed symptom, the Harvard physicians suggested that it could provide a useful early indicator for endometriosis, helping people to get treatment earlier.

The connection between endometriosis and acne is thought to be genetic as a mutation on chromosome 8q24 has been linked to a four-fold increase in the risk of severe teenage acne, and expression of a gene also on this chromosome has been linked to endometriosis. While genes themselves can't be changed, the expression and influence of genes can be modified to some extent through diet and lifestyle. The researchers also noted that changes in sex hormones, or immune malfunction, may also be involved in the development of endometriosis and acne.

Turning Things Around

Eating a low glycaemic load diet, reducing stress, and getting adequate exercise are all ways to help balance hormonal fluctuations linked to acne flare-ups.

There is some evidence that phytoestrogens, such as isoflavones from soy and lignans from flaxseed, can stimulate SHBG synthesis, thus helping to control levels of circulating androgens. A handful of studies support this theory by showing that soy and flax consumption led to increased urinary excretion of phytoestrogens over a 4-12 week period (Low et al., 2007; Pino et al., 2000; Tham et al., 1998).

In one study, women who followed a vegetarian diet had significant increases in their levels of SHBG over two menstrual cycles, compared to their SHBG levels over another two cycles (Barnard et al., 2000).

Eating organic foods and avoiding other potential sources of endocrine disruption may also play a role in keeping acne at bay. This includes minimising exposure to chemicals such as bisphenol-A, which is found in drinking bottles and food cans, and parabens found in toiletries and personal care products. As oily fish tend to concentrate endocrine-disrupting chemicals, those hoping to cure their acne by eating a diet high in omega-3 may actually find that their acne worsens through increased hormone disruption unless they opt for plant-based sources of omega-3, such as algal oil, flax and chia seeds.

A variety of other nutrients found in plant foods can also help with hormonal balance by supporting the timely detoxification and elimination of excess hormones. Such nutrients include folate, molybdenum, magnesium, and vitamin B6. Vitamin B12 is also necessary for many such processes and requires special attention as it is not naturally present in plant-based diets. B12 is often present in fortified foods however, and can be taken in supplemental form. For more on the importance of vitamin B12 in plant-based diets, check out www.veganhealth.org/articles/vitaminb12.

Practical Steps:

To help fight insulin resistance and reduce the likelihood of developing metabolic syndrome it is wise to reduce consumption of highly refined carbohydrates, such as:

- White bread, crackers, and pasta
- Baked goods using white flour
- Foods sweetened with sugar, maltose, dextrose, and other simple sugars.

Avoiding, or cutting down on these foods can help prevent rapid elevations in blood glucose that, over time, contribute to insulin resistance.

Fruit is also high in sugar, and so it may appear, at first glance, to make sense to remove fruit from the diet as well as other forms of sugar. Indeed, although fructose (the sugar found in fruit) has a low GI, it is used to induce insulin resistance in animal models of diabetes, and a similar effect is observed in humans when fructose forms 20% of calorie intake.

However, most servings of fruit contain less than 10g of carbohydrate and are a good source of soluble fibre, which slows down sugar absorption. Fresh fruits are also a fantastic source of many phytonutrients and antioxidants known to help protect skin health. So, eating some fresh fruit, but not making it a substantial part of the diet seems to be the most sensible approach, in addition to avoiding refined fructose products, such as high fructose corn syrup.

It is also a good idea to choose fresh fruit over dried fruit or fruit juice as the latter two concentrate the fructose and/or contain little if any fibre to slow down its release. This is one of the reasons why juice detox regimens often backfire; they contain a lot of sugar and barely any fibre!

In addition to looking at fruit in the diet, it is a good idea to eat at least one serving of pulses a day, such as lentils, beans, split peas, or houmous. These provide a source of low GI complex carbohydrates, protein, and fibre as well as an array of other important nutrients.

Avoiding (dairy) milk is also sensible as it is high in sugar (lactose) and often contains hormones that promote rapid weight gain and insulin resistance, as well as disrupting endogenous hormone production.

A few additional 'cheats' to help lower the GI of a meal include adding lemon juice, vinegar, or tomato sauce to foods as well as learning a few handy substitutions of low GI foods for higher GI staples:

- Try pumpernickel, oat, and sourdough instead of bread made with white or heavily refined flour.
- Choose sweet potatoes or yams instead of white potatoes (and leave the skins on!).
- Make a risotto with barley, quinoa, or even brown rice instead of white, Arborio rice.
- Switch your sugary, instant cereals for wholegrain cereals such as muesli and unsweetened granola.
- Ditch the 'low fat' versions of foods and go for regular non-dairy products.
- Soak and cook your own beans and pulses - tinned versions are often overcooked and have a lower GI.

CHAPTER THREE: IS THERE ANY TRUTH TO THESE SKIN MYTHS?

When you're battling with acne, many people will offer you advice in the form of a sure-fire acne cure. Oddly enough, none of those cures will ever have been tested, patented, and marketed and none will have helped to banish blemishes forever. Most of the time that's because these natural remedies either don't work or work so briefly as to be inconsequential to serious acne sufferers. Meanwhile, skin myths abound that link acne to chocolate, smoking, alcohol, make-up, and even under-washing or over-washing your face.

What's going on? Is there any truth to these skin myths?

In this chapter we'll examine a few of the most common skin myths and explore the reasoning and science behind them.

Myth Number One:

Smoking causes acne

Dietary changes can have a dramatic effect on healing and acne prevention, but some people also claim that quitting smoking cured their acne, so is there a link between lighting up and breaking out?

The chemicals found in tobacco smoke include carbon monoxide, which causes vasoconstriction (narrowing of the blood vessels). This decreases oxygen delivery to skin cells, causing the smaller blood vessels and capillaries near the skin's surface to dilate in order to increase blood flow and oxygenation. Over time the permanent dilation of these blood vessels causes them to become weak, resulting in broken capillaries visible on the surface of the skin. The appearance of these broken blood vessels is reminiscent of rosacea and the flushed appearance often associated with alcoholism. In addition to being surrounded by inflammation, these broken blood vessels leave the skin vulnerable to infection from bacteria associated with acne.

Smoking also reduces the amount of vitamin C available to support skin health, which could contribute to acne in a number of ways. For example, suboptimal vitamin C can lead to a higher degree of free radical damage and a reduced ability to heal the skin.

Vitamin C is essential for the production of collagen, the major structural protein that supports the skin. This is one of the reasons why smokers tend to develop wrinkles earlier than non-smokers. Another reason is that smoking impairs circulation, meaning that the skin is unable to get the nutrients and oxygen it needs to fuel repair and growth. Poor circulation also means that the skin is unable to effectively remove metabolic waste and toxins. Such effects increase the risk of acne and scarring.

The horrible irony is that smokers may turn to skin-resurfacing treatments to reduce visible acne scarring only to find that smoking makes them ineligible for treatment. That's because physicians may decide that the risk of a smoker not healing properly outweighs the potential benefits. Smokers often notice that even minor blemishes may leave scars, giving smokers an added incentive to kick the habit.

What's the VERDICT? TRUE!

Myth Number Two:

Chocolate can trigger acne breakouts

Diet and acne have been strange bed-fellows for a number of years, with myriad myths connecting spots to food choices. In most cases there is little evidence in support of the idea that foods such as chocolate increase acne, so why does the myth persist?

The problem is that excessive chocolate consumption is often linked to a generally unhealthy diet full of fat and sugar and low in wholefoods, vitamins, minerals, and phytonutrients. In some cases, chocolate consumption may also be linked to lifestyle factors including smoking, drinking, and inadequate exercise, as well as to increased stress (chocolate is a classic comfort food!). This all means that a diet high in chocolate may result in the skin (and the rest of the body) not getting the nutrition it needs to be healthy.

Blaming the chocolate doesn't really make sense, then, especially as many acne sufferers are actually reacting to the fat, dairy, and sugar in chocolate. Studies comparing carob and chocolate lend some support to this idea, as do studies that have noted flare-ups of acne, eczema, or even psoriasis in those who are intolerant or allergic to dairy.

Dairy and excess sugar in chocolate can also have a negative effect on hormone balance which, as we know from chapter two, can trigger acne. We'll look at the dairy-acne connection in more depth in chapter four.

What's the VERDICT? Partly TRUE (depending on the chocolate!)

Myth Number Three:

Using heavy make-up makes acne worse

When a pimple appears, it may be tempting to use a concealer and other kinds of make-up to mask the zit. However, relying on make-up to cover skin blemishes can, unfortunately, increase the likelihood of future skin problems. This is because make-up can block pores, affect skin moisture levels, and introduce toxins to the skin. So what can you do to make sure your make-up isn't simply perpetuating pimples?

One key thing is to always make sure to remove your make-up before going to bed as this lets the skin breathe and rest overnight. Use a gentle cleanser and toner but make sure not to scrub at your face as this can inflame the skin and make acne more likely to develop. Often, some simple olive oil on a cotton pad can easily remove make-up. Alternatively, an easy cleanser can be made by processing fresh cucumber and cold green tea in a blender (check chapter eight for more skin solution from your pantry).

Another way to reduce the negative impact of make-up on skin health is to choose noncomedogenic make-up. This is a form of make-up which doesn't block pores as much and therefore allows the skin to continue removing toxins and debris such as dead skin cells that may otherwise cause infection and acne.

Old make-up can harbour bacteria, so replacing make-up regularly can also help prevent acne, as can washing make-up applicators and brushes once or twice a week with an antibacterial soap. Alternatively, an isopropyl alcohol spray can also help decontaminate them, or you can always use disposable applicators such as cotton buds to help reduce the risk of reintroducing bacteria to your skin.

Other good ideas include using a powder-based foundation rather than an oil-based formula as the former is thought less likely to upset the moisture balance of the skin. If you have excessively oily skin then powders may in fact help soak up some of the oil and reduce acne. In addition to switching from liquid foundation to powder you may simply wish to look into a different brand. There are many cruelty-free brands out there (look for the leaping bunny logo) and some people find that a change in brand can significantly reduce their acne, possibly because of sensitivity to a particular ingredient in a formula.

It's also a good idea to have make-up-free days. This can benefit both your wallet and your skin, as well as your self-esteem because, while make-up can be fun and playful, sometimes people get into a mindset where cosmetics are an unhealthy mask or defence against the world. If this sounds familiar, consider not wearing make-up when you're on holiday or when visiting family and see if it makes a difference as to how you interact with people, and to the health of your skin.

Make-up can, however, prove helpful in battling acne because for some people it boosts self-esteem and provides emotional and psychological benefits that then translate into reduced stress and better overall health. Research suggests that some people experience considerable emotional benefits from the use of cosmetic camouflage in coping with skin conditions, including acne (Levy & Emer, 2012).

There's certainly a balance to be struck between keeping the skin clean and clear of make-up and using make-up in such a way as to enhance psychological well-being and encourage social interaction and enjoyment of life. For those whose skin problems do appear to be connected to the use of make-up, the ideal situation would be to feel comfortable and happy without make-up. However, if forgoing make-up means sabotaging emotional health this can quickly become counterproductive. Only you can decide if the benefits of using make-up are worth the possible risk of exacerbating your acne.

What's the VERDICT? Partly TRUE!

Myth Number Four:

The contraceptive pill is the best cure for acne

Many teenage girls, as well as pre-teens and women in their twenties and thirties are prescribed the contraceptive pill as a method of controlling acne breakouts. The theory behind this is that acne is often tied to hormonal disturbance, meaning that the Pill can even things out and prevent flare-ups.

However, long-term contraceptive use, particularly from an early age, is also thought to increase the risk of breast cancer (although some studies have shown no change in this risk). Oral contraceptives also have the unfortunate effect of depleting the body of a variety of nutrients, including several B vitamins, and upsetting the copper-zinc ratio. As zinc is essential for healthy functioning of the skin, the immune system, and the healing process, any deficiency in zinc will likely result in problem skin, increased scarring, and higher risk of infection. Zinc is also important for mental health, meaning that a deficiency of the mineral may affect mood.

All in all, the contraceptive pill may help control acne for some people but it can also have negative consequences, making it preferable to figure out why hormones are unbalanced and try other ways to balance them in order to manage acne.

What's the VERDICT? FALSE!

Myth Number Five:

Spots always seem to appear before a big date

Acne can be a major cause of stress and we've probably all had the experience of getting an embarrassingly obvious spot right before a date, an interview, or even right before a wedding or birthday party. Is it just bad luck or is something else going on? As this is such an important element of skin health we're going to take an in-depth look at how stress and depression, diet, lifestyle, and acne are all interconnected.

In short… **What's the VERDICT? Often TRUE!**

And, for the extended answer, let's begin by looking at an area of research called psychodermatology.

What is Psychodermatology?

The field of psychodermatology looks at the connections between our emotions and our skin. Recent research suggests a link between acne vulgaris and depression, anxiety, and other psychological issues.

Many studies don't examine which came first, the acne or the depression, but some have found that therapies to help patients feel happier actually objectively improve the condition of the skin. Conversely, finding the root cause of acne and addressing it can not only lead to healthier looking skin but also a healthier outlook on life.

Acne can Seriously Affect Your Mental Health

Although many people without acne may dismiss the skin condition as inconsequential, research has found that people with acne have a higher rate of serious mental health issues than those with other chronic, non-psychiatric medical conditions. Acne sufferers tend to be more depressed, anxious and even have higher levels of schizophrenia and psychosis than those with diabetes and epilepsy. In one study, people with acne were reported to have more emotional disability than people with asthma, epilepsy, back pain, and arthritis (Mallon et al., 1999). This skin condition also appears to have a more pronounced effect on mental health than many other skin conditions, including psoriasis, eczema, and dermatitis (Gupta et al., 2014).

Why might acne affect mental health in this way? For a start, many of us strive to achieve perfection in every area of life, including appearance, meaning that every blemish can prove a barrier to social interaction, especially to exercise and sport-related activities (Loney et al., 2008). This not only makes acne sufferers more isolated but also reduces general health and fitness which then feeds depression, anxiety, and low self-esteem, creating a vicious cycle.

People who suffered with skin conditions such as acne, psoriasis, and eczema during their teens are also more likely to have experienced bullying, teasing, and taunting. It is worth noting that such teasing is not only isolated to a patient's peers, with some teenagers reporting being subjected to ridicule and derogatory remarks from health professionals (Magin et al., 2008). Anyone experiencing inappropriate care should consider finding a different physician and reporting any health care worker who behaves inappropriately to their professional board. This is not always easy, but it can make a significant difference to health to have a physician who genuinely cares about improving your quality of life.

Depression Two to Three Times Higher in Acne Sufferers

Doctors were making the connection between acne and mental health problems as far back as the middle of the twentieth century:

> *"There is no single disease which causes more psychic trauma and more maladjustment between parents and children, more general insecurity and feelings of inferiority and greater sums of psychic assessment than does acne vulgaris" (Sulzberger, 1948).*

In one study, depression was two to three times higher in those with acne than those without, and the highest rate of depression was seen in women with acne who were older than thirty-six (Uhlenhake et al., 2010). In this study, 8.8% of patients with acne reported being clinically depressed, and twice as many women than men with acne reported being depressed (10.6% of the women vs. 5.3% of the men).

The link between acne, age, and psychiatric disturbance was also noted in a study by Barrimi and colleagues (2013), who found that patients over forty years of age who used long-term corticosteroid therapy were much more likely to have some kind of psychiatric disorder alongside their skin condition.

In another study, researchers found a 34% rate of anxiety in people aged 13-25 who suffered from acne, compared to a 10% rate in people the same age suffering from seborrheic dermatitis; 38% of the acne patients also suffered from depression, with the rate higher in women than in men (Khan et al., 2001).

How do stress and depression affect the skin and why do we get spots right before that big date?

One theory regarding the stress-acne connection is that stress negatively affects the hormones which cause increased sebum production by skin cells. Excess sebum production can lead to clogged pores and the development of pimples and acne cysts as sebum clings onto dead skin cells and harbours bacteria.

Stress and other mental health issues can also adversely affect personal hygiene, the consumption of healthy foods, the development of habits such as smoking and excess alcohol consumption, and other dietary and lifestyle factors that influence skin health.

Another proposed theory is based on the finding that acne patients are at a higher risk of gastrointestinal distress and symptoms including constipation, halitosis and gastric reflux (Zhang et al., 2008). Some 13,000 adolescents were surveyed in this study by Zhang and colleagues, and the researchers found a significant correlation between acne and abdominal bloating, which can indicate dysbiosis and gastrointestinal distress.

Leaky Gut, Food Intolerances and Acne

Way back in the 1930s when Stokes and Pillsbury first proposed a unified gut-brain-skin theory, the researchers cited prior studies showing that some 40% of those with acne had low stomach acid levels (hypochlorhydria). Low stomach acid can lead to a condition called dysbiosis, where there is an overgrowth of bad bacteria and a decline in the presence of beneficial bacteria. Dysbiosis leads to an increase in the production of toxins by bad bacteria, and inflammation in the gut, causing an increase in intestinal permeability. A leaky gut then raises the risk of food sensitivities developing as antigens pass through the gut wall into the bloodstream. Symptoms of food sensitivities can include skin problems such as acne.

This gut-brain-skin connection is thought to be one of the reasons why adults can suddenly develop an allergy to previously unproblematic foods. Increased levels of circulating antigens can lead to increased systemic inflammation, creating a whole host of problems, including skin flare-ups. More than seven decades ago, these two researchers proposed the use of what we now refer to as probiotics and omega-3 in order to help counteract the stress-induced dysbiosis and inflammation. Specifically, Stokes and Pillsbury recommended *Lactobacillus acidophilus* for skin health.

So far, just one clinical trial has been published that investigated the use of *L. acidophilus* for acne. This trial involved 45 women aged 18-35 who received either probiotic supplementation, minocycline (an antibiotic), or both the probiotic and minocycline (Jung et al., 2013). The study intended to see if the tolerability of the antibiotic regime would improve if patients were simultaneously taking probiotics. However, what the researchers found was that the total lesion counts improved across all groups, with the greatest improvement seen in patients receiving both the antibiotic and probiotic. This suggests that probiotics such as *L. acidophilus* could be a useful alternative or adjunct treatment for acne.

In other research, *Staphylococcus epidermidis*, a type of bacteria found on human skin, has been seen to help fight pathogens such as *Propionibacterium acnes*, the bacterium associated with acne vulgaris (Wang et al., 2014). *S. epidermidis* does this by fermenting glycerol on the skin to create succinic acid, a substance which inhibits the growth of *P. acnes* when applied topically. No clinical trials have yet been carried out to determine if taking *S. epidermidis* internally, or applying the friendly bacteria topically could help combat acne, but it is an interesting area of research to watch.

Low Stomach Acid Levels and Skin Problems

Insufficient levels of stomach acid (hypochlorhydria) has also been reported as a possible factor that could exacerbate acne and mental health disorders. Hypochlorhydria is a significant risk factor for the development of small intestinal bacterial overgrowth (SIBO), a condition observed in around half of patients on long-term proton pump inhibitor treatment (Lombardo et al., 2010).

In some people, the symptoms of low levels of stomach acid and excess acid production can be quite similar. This has led a number of naturopaths to express concern that many of those medicated with antacids are actually in need of additional stomach acid to help their malabsorption issues. Such supplemental acid, in the form of betaine hydrochloride, could help this group of people better digest their food and free the nutrients needed for healthy skin.

Intestinal Dysbiosis and Malabsorption

Intestinal dysbiosis caused by stress (or other factors, including, ironically, antibiotics for acne) can prevent proper absorption of nutrients such as proteins, fats, carbohydrates, B vitamins and other micronutrients. As these are needed for skin health it is unsurprising that long-term problems of intestinal dysbiosis lead to acne and other skin disorders.

Dysbiosis also means an increased toxic load as bacteria produce metabolic waste and prevent the proper elimination of toxins by breaking apart bonds between toxins and substances such as glucuronic acid.

Small intestinal bacterial overgrowth (SIBO) slows down transit time in the small intestine, encouraging the overgrowth of undesirable bacteria and causing increased gut permeability.

E. coli and Skin Flare-Ups

Compared to people without acne, patients with acne vulgaris have been found to have a higher level of reactivity to bacterial endotoxins including *Escherichia coli* lipopolysaccharide in the stool (Viana et al., 2010). Acne patients also have more of these toxins in their blood, suggesting that bacterial toxins are passing through the compromised intestinal barrier, which could trigger immune system responses in these patients.

Systemic *E. coli* endotoxin has also been seen to produce depression-like behaviour in animals (Viana et al., 2010), while highly anxious people with irritable bowel syndrome have been found to have increased reactivity to this endotoxin (Liebregts et al., 2007).

Treating the Gut to Heal the Skin

What can we do, then, to calm our inner turmoil, both in the gut and the brain?

Correcting intestinal dysbiosis typically involves the use of probiotics and antimicrobial treatment. These have been shown to help restore the integrity of the intestinal barrier, which, in turn, can improve emotional health (Pimentel et al., 2000; Addolorato et al., 2008). Correcting SIBO through the use of antibiotics led to significant improvements in rosacea in patients in one study (Parodi et al., 2008), which could mean that this skin condition would also benefit from restored intestinal eubiosis (bacterial balance).

Managing Acne Linked to Stress

As stress can upset digestive health and lead to dysbiosis, it would make sense that acne lesions are more likely to arise when a person is under excessive stress and/or when digestive health is compromised. Could this mean that talking therapies and counselling might work to reduce acne symptoms?

Stress, overwork, fatigue and skin problems go hand in hand but the connection is far more complex than simply improving your diet, making healthy lifestyle choices and getting more sleep. Many skin conditions are affected by mental health issues beyond stress, and some appear to be significantly associated with a range of psychological disorders.

Depression and skin disorders play a game of chicken and egg it seems, with skin serotonin levels influencing psoriasis and psoriasis influencing systemic inflammation and depressive markers. It's not as simple as saying that poor skin is responsible for patients' depression and it may even be the other way around for many.

More recently, researchers found that, compared to other skin disorders, acne was over two times more likely to be present in those with Attention Deficit Hyperactivity Disorder (ADHD) (Gupta et al., 2014).

Psychological Interventions for Acne

Psychotherapy, and the promotion of self-insight, has been shown to have long-term benefits for many patients, but it has rarely been studied for its usefulness in cases of acne (Gray, 1990; Blatt & Behrends, 1987). Controlled studies have however, noted remarkable improvements with the use of biofeedback techniques, and a combination of biofeedback, relaxation training, and cognitive behavioral therapy (Hughes et al., 1983).

Cognitive behavioural therapy can also help us kick some unhealthy habits, such as picking at pimples. Pimple-picking is frowned upon by dermatologists everywhere, but these skin specialists also know that they cannot simply prescribe 'leaving your pimples alone' as an acne remedy, despite it being sage advice.

Stress can make us fidgety and increase behaviours such as pulling at the hair, twiddling pens, chewing pencils, tapping our feet or picking at our spots. Picking at acne blemishes increases the risks of skin infection and scarring and also spreads the bacteria to other parts of the skin, creating a chain reaction of acne when stressed. Addressing acne may, in rare cases, be as simple as taking the time to meditate and avoiding touching the face with your hands. For most people, however, it will take a little more work to resolve psychodermatological issues underlying acne.

There have been numerous calls over recent years to take psychological health into account when devising a treatment strategy for acne (Layton, 2001). Not only is it preferable to treat acne early and try to prevent scarring, it is also advisable to consider the emotional impact of acne and scarring and therefore incorporate psychological therapy into treatment plans for acne.

There have been reports of acne clearing up with the use of antidepressants in some patients with both acne and depression, although symptoms typically return when medications are discontinued. Clearly, anyone prescribed antidepressants by their physician should avoid making changes to their medications without consultation.

The use of a technique known as eye movement desensitization and reprocessing (EMDR) has also shown benefit for several dermatological conditions, including atopic dermatitis and psoriasis, and in one patient with acne excoríee, a type of acne associated with body image pathology where the patient picks at the skin due to stress and trauma (Gupta & Gupta, 2002). Marked improvements were seen in this patient with acne excoríee after 3-6 sessions of EMDR over a period of three months, with the improvement maintained after 6-12 months.

It is, therefore, a good idea for acne sufferers to discuss the use of adjunct therapies for acne that can alleviate stress and depression, thereby improving general health and well-being and increasing motivation to tackle any other causes of acne.

Practical Steps:

In addition to quitting smoking, practicing good make-up hygiene, and reassessing choices of chocolate and other possible dietary acne triggers, some basic tips for coping with skin issues include reducing the impact of stress by:

- Staying hydrated (cut out the caffeine and drink water!)
- Ensuring a good supply of magnesium, B vitamins, zinc and other important minerals and vitamins for the skin
- Considering the use of a daily probiotic to combat dysbiosis and support optimal gastrointestinal health
- Cutting out alcohol, as this increases stress responses and dehydrates the skin
- Getting quality outdoor exercise time to boost vitamin D production, endorphin levels, and circulation
- Taking time to relax!

Some natural interventions, such as omega-3 fatty acids, probiotics, chromium, folic acid, zinc, and selenium, have been seen to have benefits both for acne and mood, meaning that these may be ideal for those experiencing acne, stress, and depression (Rubin et al., 2008; Katzman & Logan, 2007).

Dietary and lifestyle modifications have been shown to help people decrease their risk of symptoms of depression and stress. However, anyone who is concerned about their mental health, including how it may be affecting acne, should be sure to consult their health care practitioner before making any changes.

CHAPTER FOUR: GOT MILK? GOT ACNE?

Chocolate has traditionally been blamed for acne flare-ups, much to the annoyance of many a teen, but there is no conclusive evidence suggesting that chocolate itself is to blame for acne. Indeed, dark chocolate may help improve skin health by increasing intake of antioxidants and arginine, an amino acid that can relax blood vessels and benefit circulation.

So why point the finger at chocolate as an acne trigger? Well, the weight of evidence suggests that it is the sugar, fat, and dairy content of milk chocolate that are really to blame.

A variety of potential mechanisms connect milk consumption to skin breakouts. Some of these possible links between dairy and acne include:

- High levels of lactose (a sugar), particularly in low-fat dairy products.
- Adverse effects of dairy on the gastrointestinal system.
- Increased inflammation from lactose intolerance.
- Dairy-induced digestive upset and impaired nutrient absorption.
- Hormones in dairy that stimulate rapid cellular growth and division.
- Abnormally high levels of some hormones, particularly testosterone, in many low-fat dairy products.
- Antibiotic and pesticide residues in milk products.
- Bacterial contamination in milk from cows with mastitis, and/or faecal contamination.
- Excess iodine in dairy.

If that list doesn't have you considering switching to a plant-based milk instead of dairy milk then I don't know what will!

Let's take a closer look at this list and see if the evidence really does stack up to support the elimination of dairy from your diet to benefit skin health and reduce acne.

Lactose Intolerance, GI Inflammation, Dysbiosis, and Acne

We've already talked about the link between acne and excess sugar consumption, but the lactose found in milk products can also trigger acne through mechanisms unrelated to a high glycaemic load diet.

Lactose intolerance is estimated to be an issue for the majority of adults as only a small percentage of people carry a mutated gene that allows for the continued production of lactase (the enzyme that breaks down lactose) into adulthood. In almost everyone else, levels of lactase decline by some 75-90% in early childhood (Newcomer et al., 1978). Indeed, in a study that looked at nine year-old children in Sardinia, some 85% had stopped producing sufficient lactase to digest milk (Schirru et al., 2007). Most adults become lactose intolerant between the ages of 20 and 40 (Kern & Struthers, 1966), and only those with northern European ancestors are thought likely to continue producing sufficient lactase to allow for reasonable digestion of milk products in adulthood (Vuorisalo et al., 2012).

This means that for most people, consuming dairy products leads to undigested lactose entering the gut, where it feeds the growth of undesirable bacteria. These bacteria can cause increased flatulence, halitosis, diarrhoea, and other unpleasant digestive disturbances commonly associated with lactose intolerance. Dairy can also cause those with lactose intolerance to experience increased levels of inflammation and problems of toxicity in the bowel as the population of bad bacteria in the gut increases and these bacteria release toxins.

Milk and other dairy produce can also impair the gut's ability to absorb nutrients, which in turn deprives the body of much-needed antioxidants and the right components to create new, healthy skin. Toxic build-up, increased inflammation, and impaired absorption of nutrients create a triple-whammy for acne sufferers eating dairy. Add to this the potential for immune system abnormalities triggered by a reaction to undigested dairy produce and you have quite the recipe for skin disease.

Standard Treatments for Acne

Rather than recommend removing dairy from the diet, the usual approach to acne is to offer palliative treatments. These often include such things as antibiotic cleansers and creams, use of oral contraceptives, steroid treatments, high doses of vitamin A, and even oral antibiotics. Such medications have the potential to cause serious health issues and, while their use may help clear up skin issues, they don't typically address the underlying problem. This means that long-term health may be adversely affected, and that stopping such treatments will result in a return of more severe acne. Antibiotics used for acne also increase the potential for antibiotic resistance, with serious consequences if an infection then occurs.

The use of antibiotics makes sense if the cause of acne is bacterial overgrowth on the skin. However, this is not the only trigger for acne. The problem, then, with the treatment of acne using antibiotics and the contraceptive pill is that these treatments also change the natural flora of the body. This dysbiosis can further exacerbate acne. In effect, the cure may become the cause.

A Gut Feeling About Acne

A significant number of studies have found strong associations between bacterial dysbiosis in the gut and stress, acne, gastrointestinal disturbance, and depression. The environment in the gut can change considerably in cases of chronic stress, causing an altered population of gastrointestinal bacteria.

Healthy gut bacteria are needed to synthesise vitamins, eliminate toxins, protect the gut wall, and carry out other essential symbiotic functions. Maintaining good bacteria in the gut, through diet and probiotics, is one way for many acne sufferers to control symptoms and keep skin healthy.

Bacterial Contamination of Dairy Products

Many people don't realise that there is a significant risk of dairy products (particularly raw, unpasteurised milk products) being contaminated with bacteria. This is partly due to the high levels of mastitis in dairy cows caused by a perpetual cycle of pregnancy and lactation. Mastitis is an infection of the milk ducts, and selective breeding and the use of growth hormones have caused an increase in risk factors for mastitis, including an incredible increase in milk production by dairy cows. Between 1940 and 2012, the average milk yield from a dairy cow went from 2 tonnes to 10 tonnes per year (US EPA, 2009).

Dairy cows are almost always housed in groups of hundreds or even thousands in milking barns where they are lined up side-by-side in filthy stalls and attached to rotating automatic milking machinery. The rate of infection in these animals is, understandably, very high and the dramatically engineered increase in milk yield has come along with serious health issues such as mastitis (USDA APHIS VS, 2007).

The automatic nature of the industry means that a cow can develop this infection without anyone noticing her pain and suffering and she will continue to be milked despite her udders being swollen and inflamed. Pus, blood, and antibodies from the infected ducts then mix with the milk during extraction and end up in the finished product, increasing the risk of bacterial infection and immune system challenges in those consuming this milk.

MRSA and Agricultural Antibiotics

Knowing that these infections are rife in their animals, the dairy and meat industry began several years ago to prophylactically treat cows. This meant adding antibiotics to their feed, rather than identifying a sick cow, giving her a break from milk production, and nurturing her back to health (USDA NASS, 2013).

It is estimated that around 90% of all antibiotics are used in animal agriculture. These antibiotics find their way into the animal foods on the average person's plate and are implicated in the development of antibiotic resistant bacterial strains that cause deadly infections (such as methicillin resistant *Staphylococcus aureus* - MRSA).

Dairy Products and Hormonal Upheaval

Acne tends to strike during the teenage years and during perimenopause; times of major hormonal upheaval. The high degree of incidence of teenage acne might suggest that it is almost a rite of passage (some surveys found that acne affects 85% of teens), but studies now show an association between dairy intake in high school and an increased risk of severe teenage acne (Adebamowo et al., 2005). Ditching the dairy and adopting a plant-based, low GI, antioxidant and anti-inflammatory rich diet may therefore help lessen the incidence and reduce the severity of acne in kids and young adults.

The interplay between the body's hormones and the skin is studied by dermatoendocrinologists. These scientists have repeatedly found that typical Western dietary patterns have a significant effect on our hormone levels, and are likely heavily involved in the pathogenesis of acne.

Milk and other dairy products increase circulating levels of insulin-like growth-factor-1 (IGF-1) by being a source of IGF-1 in themselves and by stimulating our own synthesis of IGF-1. Other factors in the Western diet, such as high fat and meat intake, high glycaemic load, and excessive calories, also increase levels of circulating IGF-1.

As we saw in chapter two, IGF-1 is a growth factor that increases protein synthesis, triggers excessive cell growth, inhibits the removal of damaged cells, and increases cell division. IGF-1 has been linked to cancer and to skin conditions involving rapid cell growth, and may increase the risk of acne by causing pores to become blocked and susceptible to infection.

Explosive Growth, Testosterone and Dairy-Acne

Cows' milk is intended to feed baby cows (naturally!) and fuel the rapid growth in calves by providing anabolic steroids, true growth hormones, and other growth factors, such as IGF-1. Human babies (and adults!) are not, however, going to grow to be the size of an adult cow and so the consumption of the milk of another species has some serious design flaws for our own physiology.

For example, milk contains the steroid hormones 5a-androstanedione, and 5alpha-pregnanedione (5alpha-P) which are direct precursors of 5a-dihydrotestosterone, a hormone associated with prostate cancer development (Danby, 2010). Epidemiological research links dairy consumption not only with acne and prostate cancer, but also with breast cancer as 5alpha-P increases sensitivity to oestrogen in breast tissue (Danby, 2009).

We produce some dihydrotestosterone ourselves but by consuming ready-made exogenous hormones and growth factors in dairy products and meat it may be that we begin to overwhelm our carefully evolved feedback systems, leading to rapid cell growth (hyperplasia or neoplasia).

Dairy Consumption and Oily Skin

Melnik (2012) also noted that dairy can increase levels of circulating hormones and IGF-1, in part by activating mTORC1 (mammalian target of rapamycin complex 1), which is responsible for cellular energy signalling. Too much mTORC1 results in excessive creation of lipids, especially by sebocytes, leading to oily skin and the potential for pores to become blocked, triggering acne. Over-activated mTORC1 also increases androgen hormone synthesis, which again activates sebaceous follicles.

Testosterone directly activates mTORC1, meaning that the testosterone found naturally in animal products can lead to excessive lipogenesis (synthesis of fats in the body), increased fat, oily skin, and, potentially, acne. Plants do not contain testosterone and, instead, can help regulate hormone levels due to their fibre content and possible phytoestrogen effects.

Acne: A 'Disease of Civilisation'

Meat and dairy also contain high amounts of leucine, an amino acid that increases mTORC1 activity. Melnik (2012) considers epidemic acne to be an "mTORC1 driven disease of civilization like obesity, type 2 diabetes, cancer and neurodegenerative diseases." The suggestion, then, is that avoiding consumption of dairy, meat and other hormone-disrupting, mTORC1-activating factors, could reduce the incidence of these diseases, including acne.

Melnik goes as far as to recommend that dermatologists advise acne patients to adopt a vegan diet that emphasises vegetables and fruit, in order to reduce mTORC1 stimulation and improve skin health and a number of other health parameters.

Dietary Improvements for Acne Eradication

One case-controlled study looked at the relationship between a high glycaemic load diet, milk and ice cream consumption and the incidence and severity of acne vulgaris in young adults aged 18-30 (Ismail et al., 2012). The 44 participants filled out a questionnaire detailing family history and dietary patterns and were asked to keep a record of their food intake for two weekdays and one weekend day. They were assessed by a dermatologist for acne severity using the comprehensive acne severity scale (CASS).

The results showed that those with more severe acne had a considerably higher glycaemic load, consumed milk and ice cream much more often than the controls, and that the differences were most significant in the women in the study.

Despite the stark support from this study of a link between dairy and acne, more studies are needed as this was a small, short study, reliant on participants' accuracy in recording food intake. Fortunately, other studies do substantiate this link between dairy and acne.

Skim Milk Almost Doubles Acne Risk!

One piece of high-quality evidence comes courtesy of a retrospective analysis using data from the Nurses Health Study II (Adebamowo et al., 2005). In this research, scientists looked at the reported intake of dairy foods during high school and found a significant association with physician-diagnosed severe teenage acne. Some 47,355 women completed questionnaires on high school diet and, after accounting for age, age at menarche, Body Mass Index, and energy intake, acne prevalence in the women increased by:

- 22% for excessive milk intake
- 12% for whole milk
- 16% for low-fat milk
- 44% for skim milk.

Instant breakfast drink, sherbet, cottage cheese, and cream cheese were also positively associated with acne.

These results suggest that low-fat milk is particularly likely to increase the incidence of acne. This is likely because of the higher concentration of both lactose (milk sugar) and hormones in milk that has been processed to remove fat. The removal of fat also means that the milk sugars will be broken down more quickly, increasing blood sugar and leading to a higher requirement for insulin production. As we saw in previous chapters, higher levels of dietary sugar can increase insulin resistance, metabolic syndrome and subsequent acne.

One of the Easiest Ways to Reduce Acne Risk

A plant-based diet clearly has no room for milk products, but you might be wondering what effect eggs could have on your skin. Despite being a good source of many nutrients vital for skin health, eggs are also a significant dietary source of sex hormones which can upset our own hormonal balance (Hartmann et al., 1998). They are also susceptible to many of the same issues as with milk, including antibiotic and pesticide residues, and bacterial contamination.

Are soy milk, almond milk, coconut or cashew milk any better for your skin? If you think back to the last chapter, where we talked about hormones, metabolic syndrome, and skin health, you might recall that soy appears to have properties that could help improve at least one cause of acne, namely hormone disturbances. For those whose acne is connected to polycystic ovary syndrome (PCOS) and low levels of sex hormone binding globulin (SHBG), soy and flaxseed may offer some assistance by boosting levels of SHBG and helping to bring unruly hormones back under control.

These plant-based milks contain numerous nutrients necessary for healthy skin, including calcium, monounsaturated and polyunsaturated fatty acids, B vitamins, magnesium, zinc, and protein. It's best to choose organic, unsweetened versions of non-dairy milks though, in order to avoid pesticide residues and increased inflammation from excess dietary sugars.

Practical Steps

Most people are brought up with the idea that milk and dairy products are the key to good health. This means that most people have never experienced life without these food staples and therefore have no idea what it feels like to live without systemic, low-grade symptoms of lactose intolerance, dysbiosis, and other sources of ill-health. This also means that it can be hard to imagine a diet without milk and dairy products, and it's certainly not recommended to rapidly eliminate a major source of calories and nutrients without having a firm idea of how to replace those things with healthier options.

The best approach is to start slow by taking stock of the sources of dairy in your diet. This means the milk on your cereal, the cream in your coffee, the butter on your bread, and all the 'hidden' dairy elsewhere in foods. If you've tried to cut out dairy before and had little to show for it then it's important to realise that removing the obvious culprits might not be enough. If your acne is tied to dairy consumption then it is necessary to acknowledge how frequently dairy derivatives turn up as ingredients in processed foods and to find dairy-free alternatives.

Many people fall into the trap of simply cutting out milk and cheese only to find that their skin is still covered in blemishes. Cutting out all dairy can take a bit of time and practice and it's wise to make a pact with yourself to be forgiving if you slip up every now. It's not an all or nothing game, so finding out that the slice of bread you just ate, or the soup you had for lunch contains dairy doesn't mean that it makes sense to go and eat a triple cheese pizza for dinner.

Easy switches to make include:

- Using soy, almond, oat, coconut, rice, or hemp milk for your morning granola and cup of tea
- Asking for soy or coconut creamer for your coffee (most chain coffee shops have these)
- Buying dairy-free cheese shreds for sandwich fillings or using vegan mayo, guacamole, or houmous instead
- Ordering your pizza without cheese or asking the restaurant if they have a vegan cheese substitute on hand (many do!)

Once you start feeling a bit more comfortable with some favourite vegan pantry items you can expand your dairy-free culinary range and think about:

- Making pizza at home and using a sprinkling of nutritional yeast instead of cheese as a topping
- Grinding up Brazil nuts, salt, nutritional yeast and a dash of hemp oil to make dairy-free parmesan
- Adding coconut or cashew cream to soups
- Making tofu cashew ricotta as a baked potato filling
- Making macadamia and cashew 'goat's' cheese

The likelihood is that any food you're craving that's dairy-based has already been 'veganised' by someone and may even have a commercially available substitute. The beauty of cutting out dairy is that it often makes you much more aware of what's in your food, allowing you to make fresh, nutritious, whole food versions at home.

CHAPTER 5: DO CLEANSES REALLY WORK FOR SPOT-PRONE SKIN?

"Long-term fasts lead to muscle breakdown and a shortage of many needed nutrients... [which can] actually weaken the body's ability to fight infections and inflammation."

Lona Sandon, RD. and spokesperson for the American Dietetic Association.

Clearer skin is one of the many purported benefits of juice cleanses, the so-called Master Cleanse, and other detoxification regimes, but is there anything of substance to these fad diets? Could they actually be harmful and make acne worse?

'Detox' diets are common fodder for headlines, with a multitude of celebrities extolling the virtues of one cleanse or another. However, we are not all celebrities looking to quickly drop twenty pounds for a movie role, with a dedicated medical team to ensure our safety and help us rebuild the lost muscle mass afterwards. Indeed, Beyoncé, who used the Master Cleanse to prepare for her role in Dreamgirl has openly admitted that it can be harmful and that she would never have done it without such assistance or for anything other than that role.

Why Are Cleanses Popular?

Cleanses are touted as a way of removing harmful toxins from the body as well as for:

- Promoting weight loss
- Refreshing the appearance of the skin

- Regulating digestion
- Boosting the immune system
- Improving mental clarity
- Strengthening libido.

It's easy to see why a cleanse may seem ideal if you're feeling sluggish and unhealthy after eating a lot of rich foods and consuming a lot of alcohol. It's also the case that many people with a newly diagnosed health condition begin to think about doing regular cleanses, while others may consider cleanses to help combat persistent acne.

Whatever the motivation for detoxing, the key is to harness that energy and send it in a healthy direction, which doesn't necessitate a three-day juice fast or Master Cleanse.

Do We Really Need to Detox?

Unsurprisingly, given so many years of evolution, our bodies are actually pretty good at removing harmful substances and detoxifying toxins. This means that for many people the cycle of 'indulgence' and 'detox' is based on guilt rather than good science. In the case of acne, there may be an element of feeling somehow 'unclean' because of skin blemishes, leading to a desire to undergo a cleanse in part for its psychological value.

The truth is that we are exposed to a vast array of environmental toxins daily, and that we also produce our own toxins through the normal processes of metabolism. For example, we are consistently exposed to heavy metals in our water, food, beauty products, cooking utensils, and even medications, along with hormone-disrupting chemicals found in plastics, clothing, toiletries, food, water, and, again, medications.

Rather than relying on the occasional extreme cleanse to rid us of these, it makes much more sense to limit our exposure to toxins and to bolster the body's ability to safely process and eliminate these chemicals.

Spring-Cleaning the Body

To demonstrate the benefits of forming consistently healthy habits, consider the scenario where you decide one day to simply leave all household chores until spring and then do a 'house detox.' Come spring, you'll realise that you've spent all year being grumpy and sick due to living in squalor, and that you now need to put in a gargantuan amount of effort to clean all those dishes, scrub the floors, wash the bedding, and remove all that nasty gunk from the plughole. If you'd simply taken care of things as they arose, keeping things orderly and clean, you could have had an enjoyable year and still have a lot of energy to put towards fun things.

To stretch out the metaphor, if you did take on this arduous task of cleaning up your neglected house then you'd likely run out of detergent, time, money, and energy before everything was ship-shape. This is really no different to how your body functions, and demonstrates one of the ways in which detoxes are doomed. It takes a lot more energy to eliminate built-up toxins from a sluggish and unhealthy system than it does to clean as you go, while energy levels are consistent. If your chosen cleanse is extremely low calorie then it's also highly likely that you'll get pretty tired pretty quickly.

And, if you do opt for a dramatic cleanse, even while you're cleaning and scrubbing to try to get on top of things again, more dirty plates, trash, and recycling are piling up. When applied to the skin, this means that your skin's cells are struggling to replicate properly to facilitate healing, excess oil may start blocking the pores, and abnormal cellular changes or processes may occur leading to scarring, pigment problems, and even skin cancer.

The temptation to let things slide for most of the year and then spend three days drinking nothing but lemon juice and cayenne pepper is clear but, as with so many things in life, the key to healthy skin and overall health is accepting a certain reality. That reality is that you need to be pretty consistent about making healthy choices and avoiding exposure to toxins if you don't want the junk to pile up.

Common Toxins

Potential toxins are all around us in the form of rancid fats, fungus, oxidised proteins, petrochemicals, viruses and mould. While it's impossible to avoid all sources of these, we can certainly do our best to minimise exposure and keep the body in good shape so as to deal with the potential insults from such toxins.

Reducing exposure to undesirable chemicals can involve switching to natural bodycare products, choosing fresh whole foods, buying clothing and furnishings made using organic cotton and other fabrics, and using cooking utensils made of cast iron, glass, and ceramics that don't contain bisphenol-A, plasticisers, and other nasty endocrine disruptors.

Types of Cleanse

Having said all this, let's have a look at two types of popular cleanse and how these claim to help acne and other conditions.

The 'Master Cleanse' - Drinking fresh lemon juice, sugar or maple syrup, and cayenne pepper for ten days in place of all other food except black tea.

The reasoning: The Master Cleanse was developed in the 1940s by a chap called Stanley Burroughs and got a second wind in the 1970s with his book *The Master Cleanser*. The diet is a modified juice fast that is supposed to help detoxify the body and remove excess fat.

The reality: There is no evidence to support these claims and it is actually much more likely to lead to rapid loss of water weight and muscle mass rather than fat. This ends up making it harder to rebuild lost muscle and more likely that a person will gain weight in the form of fat. As the diet lacks protein, the longer it is maintained the more muscle is lost and the more muscle healing is impaired. As the heart is a muscle it suffers a double-whammy with this type of cleanse, losing strength while also being adversely affected by electrolyte imbalances.

This 'diet' is deficient in protein, vitamins, minerals, fats, and calories in general which can lead to symptoms of fatigue, nausea, dizziness, and dehydration. Those with existing health issues may suffer more significantly if they try the Master Cleanse. In particular, those with heart issues, poor blood glucose control, elevated stress levels, and even mental health issues such as depression are at a higher risk of complications even in the short term. This diet deprives the body of practically everything it needs to function well and to deal with toxins in a healthy way.

The negative effects of this diet on stress hormones, blood sugar control, healing processes and detoxification mechanisms is actually more likely to trigger skin breakouts and impair the health of the skin in regards to scarring and abnormal cellular processes. A hunger-induced euphoria and placebo effect may convince some of the short-term benefits for acne and weight loss but this 'cleanse' is unhelpful over the long-term and may be dangerous.

A seven-day juice cleanse - Replacing all meals and snacks with juices made from (preferably organic) fruits and vegetables.

The reasoning: This kind of cleanse is said to free our bodies of the need to expend energy digesting solid food and so give us spare energy to pull toxins from the cells and tissues and detoxify and eliminate those toxins, leading to clearer, brighter skin. Juice cleanses do away with the fibre component of fruits and vegetables, meaning that followers can consume higher quantities of juice and, therefore, more concentrated vitamins and phytonutrients to kick-start the liver and kidneys and flush toxins out of the body.

The reality: By doing away with the fibre, the sugar content of these foods is much more concentrated. This can lead to hyperglycaemia, insulin resistance and pre-diabetes, hormone disruption, inflammation, and worse acne.

Such juice fasts are also woefully lacking in fats and proteins, which means that many fat soluble vitamins (A, D, E, and K) are unable to be properly absorbed or used in the body.

Additionally, while fruits and vegetables are great sources of antioxidants and other beneficial compounds, they are not generally very good sources of minerals such as selenium and zinc, or vitamins E, D, B12, and other B vitamins. This lack of nutrients, especially protein, impairs healing and immune system function.

Many popular cleanses are short-lived, lasting around three to ten days, and so are unlikely to cause long-term vitamin and mineral deficiency symptoms. However, water soluble vitamins are not stored in the body and are therefore needed daily, meaning that signs of insufficiency can arise quite quickly.

An acute lack of B vitamins can, for example, cause problems with sleep and with our ability to handle stress, as well as adversely affecting hormonal balance and digestion. Juice fasts are extremely stressful to the body and, as we saw in chapter three, increased stress is a major factor in many cases of acne, as is hormonal imbalance.

Cleanses as Stressors - Why We Get a Juice-Fast 'Buzz'

Juice cleanses often involve the consumption of incredible amounts of simple sugars in the form of fructose, which not only leads to a sugar-high, but also to insulin resistance, and acne.

In addition to the spikes in blood sugar, the energy rush many feel in the middle of a detox may be attributed to increased levels of cortisol and adrenaline. These hormones are produced by the body in response to stressors, such as feeling that it is being starved. That juice-fast 'buzz' may simply be your body telling you to hunt and gather some proper food.

A spate of spotty skin during a detox is often explained away as a sign that the toxins are leaving your system. In fact, it's actually more likely that your juice cleanse is proving extremely stressful to your body, disrupting your hormones, and spiking your blood sugar, leading to acne flare-ups.

Nutrients and Detoxification

There may be times when complete removal of a specific food or food group from the diet is warranted, but this is usually only in cases of diagnosed or suspected allergy or intolerance, or when food is known to be contaminated in some way. The reality is that when we eat fresh fruits, vegetables, whole grains, nuts, seeds, legumes, pulses, and other healthy whole foods, we're actually 'cleansing' all the time. These foods give us the minerals, vitamins, water, and energy, along with phytonutrients, that we need to effectively disable toxins and flush them from the body.

A specific example of this is the mineral zinc which is needed for hundreds of enzyme reactions in the body. Zinc-dependent enzymes are involved in skin cell production and healthy healing and immunity as well as elimination of heavy metals. Dangerous metals such as cadmium, mercury, and lead may enter our systems through old water pipes, medications, and contaminated food (particularly foods from animals higher up in the food chain, where toxins are concentrated).

When we have insufficient amounts of zinc and other co-factors for detoxification it is difficult for the body to safely and promptly eliminate heavy metals and prevent cellular damage. Those who are deficient in zinc are also more susceptible to the absorption of cadmium in the gut, as well as to its negative effects on the body after it has been absorbed (Brzóska & Moniuszko-Jakoniuk, 2001).

There are many more examples of minerals that are essential for certain detoxification enzymes to function, including selenium, on which the GPx enzyme relies, and CAT which relies on iron. One key detoxification enzyme, superoxide dismutase (SOD), is dependent on zinc, copper and manganese. As such, any detox diet lacking these nutrients could be accused of actively working against normal and healthy detoxification processes.

When a diet is unbalanced in terms of any one of these nutrients required for detoxification there is a weightier burden on the other nutrients, meaning that even a diet that appears to have adequate zinc may, on balance, be insufficient if selenium and manganese are lacking. As zinc is so vital for skin health and so strongly associated with acne development and outbreaks it is easy to see why a cleanse that provides suboptimal levels of this mineral (and its co-factors in detoxification) can prove so damaging for the skin.

Why Toxins Are Bad, but Cleanses May be Worse

Daily exposure to toxins, and poor detoxification processes, can lead to a weakened immune system and inflammation. In turn, weakened immunity can increase the risk of acne by allowing bacterial overgrowth on the skin and in the gut. Unchecked inflammation, meanwhile, can cause blemishes to appear more pronounced and swollen and result in lingering tissue damage.

Sadly, many people looking for a 'quick fix' through a juice cleanse or other detox regime already have compromised health, and it is precisely this group of people for whom detox diets can be especially dangerous.

Of course, there are times where detoxification really is impaired, such as in people with organ dysfunction and disease. Patients may require dialysis, a kidney transplant, or a liver transplant, or the long-term use of certain medications to help support normal bodily processes. Following physician advice regarding detoxification is vital in such cases.

Specific dietary practices may be helpful for those whose ability to detoxify is compromised, such as reducing intake of fats or avoiding eating meals combining sources of calcium with sources of oxalic acid. These situations are relatively rare, however, with most people consistently able to manage the detoxification and elimination of undesirable compounds and substances. If you suspect that you have a serious issue with regards to detoxification then it is vital to seek medical attention from a qualified professional as a cleanse could do more harm than good and land you in hospital with heart palpitations, gut perforation, or kidney failure.

Cleanses for Body, Mind, and Soul.

Anyone who is feeling run down, depressed, stressed, unlovable, and acne-prone may be tempted to try an extreme cleanse. Unfortunately, these cleanses can not only make acne worse, they may lead to increased fatigue and infections as well as an increased vulnerability to stress and depression.

Taking steps to better overall health for mind and body, as a consistent way of life, offers a much better approach that can provide good long-term outcomes. If a cleanse looks tempting then it may be helpful to consider your motivations, and what you hope to gain from such a regimen. That way, you can prioritise your goals and find healthier ways to achieve them that don't put you at risk.

Of course, discussing detox diets and cleanses means getting bogged down in semantics as what one person sees as a cleanse is actually an everyday diet for someone else. Some 'cleanses' can, therefore, have benefits for acne and overall health.

A cleanse that involves a permanent switch to a more healthful whole food, plant-based diet devoid of many of the most obvious sources of toxins, hormone-disrupters and simple sugars is likely to be of benefit for the skin. In addition to the direct benefits of switching to this kind of diet, recognising that you are making such healthy changes can itself induce positive effects on your skin, energy levels, and happiness.

When you feel that it is worth looking after yourself then you are more likely to sleep well, avoid excessive alcohol consumption, quit smoking, exercise regularly, and practice healthier lifestyle and dietary habits in general. It may be a bit of a catch-22, that you need to have self-worth in order to treat yourself as valuable but that's where a healthy diet masquerading as a cleanse may help. By adopting a healthy regimen, even in the short-term, a person may find that it becomes a way of life and that these new foods and practices are more sustainable and rewarding than they had imagined. In effect, the placebo becomes the cure.

Before we wrap up this chapter on detoxification, let's take a moment to highlight some things to watch out for with cleanses.

If It Quacks....

Any cleanse or detox diet that necessitates you buying a mysterious, rare, elusive product from a specific source should be approached with caution. There is no magic pill, juice, plant extract, or other product that will single-handedly eradicate toxins from the body.

There are certainly many natural substances that have potent antioxidant activity and enzyme-activating properties that can form a useful part of a normal routine. Including such natural substances can support the body in dealing with unavoidable exposure to toxins.

However, anyone touting a magic bullet for detoxification should be regarded with intense scepticism.

> *"Stay away from weird dietary practices. If they sound weird, they are."*
>
> **Marion Nestle, Professor of Nutrition, Food Studies, and Public Health at New York University and author of What to Eat (2007).**

Colon-Cleanses and Constipation

Those espousing the benefits of more extreme spa procedures such as colon-cleanses often claim that these methods work as a quick-fix detox. Unsurprisingly, there is a distinct lack of evidence to support these claims, and, in fact, colon cleanses may prove harmful as they can adversely affect electrolyte balance and flush out the beneficial bacteria necessary for a healthy gut.

Colonic irrigation can also flush out both good and bad bacteria in the gut, leading to problems connected to dysbiosis. In addition to dysbiosis-related issues such as increased inflammation, immune system dysfunction, and impaired ability to absorb nutrients, perforation of the colon is another potential hazard of such treatments.

Other cleanses involve the prolonged use of laxatives such as Epsom salts and herbs including *Cascara sagrada* or prunes. While short-term use of these may not prove particularly harmful they can still adversely affect intestinal eubiosis and lead to bad bacterial overgrowth and infections with Candida albicans or other organisms.

If a person is constipated, there is usually a reason, meaning that simply using laxatives can ignore the underlying problem, allowing constipation to recur. A constipated colon can indicate irritation or damage in the bowel, and as strong laxatives irritate the bowel these could cause serious damage including intestinal bleeding and perforation. Long-term use of some laxatives can even reduce the capacity of the gastrointestinal tract to manage faecal elimination, making constipation a major issue and leading people to become reliant on such products for bowel movements.

Laxative products included in many cleanses may also lead to dehydration and loss of electrolytes. This may trigger abnormal heart rhythms, muscle cramps, kidney dysfunction, and confusion or other cognitive effects (another possible mechanism behind the euphoria some feel when detoxing). In addition to low blood sugar from a lack of calories, these effects may slow reaction times and make things such as driving and childcare much more dangerous.

A healthier way to cleanse the colon is to eat a healthy diet that includes adequate fibre, water, probiotics and prebiotics. It is important to ensure sufficient water intake when increasing fibre in the diet so as to avoid irritation and ensure that waste matter moves regularly through the digestive tract, cleaning the gut walls as it goes. There is no evidence that food waste sticks to the walls of the gut, making it unlikely that colonic irrigation is necessary to remove hardened toxic matter in the bowel.

Alternative 'Cleanse' - The Healthier Way

In conclusion, most cleanses and detox diets lack the basic requirements for health as recommended by dietitians, doctors, and health authorities the world over. The risks of such cleanses outweigh any potential benefits and are much more likely to trigger acne breakouts than to help you achieve clear skin. Those peddling detox diets typically rely on fear, desperation and a lack of understanding of how the body works.

As always, education is vital in protecting yourself from quacks and cranks. Learning how to nourish your skin and reduce your toxin intake and exposure can help you avoid many health issues and feel more consistently happy and energised - no dramatic detoxing needed.

CHAPTER SIX: INFLAMMATION & ACNE

In earlier chapters we have seen how acne and other skin conditions are often linked to undesirable inflammation. While inflammation is a natural and helpful response to an injury or infection, chronic inflammation is a significant contributing factor in many illnesses. Inflammation and swelling that continues over weeks, months, or even years is abnormal and needs attention.

Prematurely quashing an inflammatory reaction to injury or infection can impair the body's ability to cope with these events, possibly even preventing wounds from properly closing, or encouraging the spread of an isolated infection. Additionally, some degree of muscle inflammation is actually necessary for muscle growth, and many sports physiotherapists now recognise that applying ice and administering anti-inflammatory drugs too quickly after muscle strain may actually delay healing and recovery. The trick is determining just how long to let normal inflammatory processes go unchecked and when to step in to combat problematic persistent inflammation.

Acute and chronic trauma and irritation can increase localised inflammation. Trauma and irritation in the skin can result from:

- Aggressive scrubbing
- Overuse of exfoliating products
- Use of cleansers with a high alcohol content
- Use of lotions containing:
  - fragrance
  - preservatives
  - lanolin (which is derived from sheep fat)
  - parabens
  - EDTA (Ethylenediaminetetraacetic acid)

- mineral oil (a by-product of gasoline production).

Choosing natural skin products that are free of these common irritants can help reduce the incidence and severity of acne. It is also advisable to choose products which actively soothe inflammation and help the skin retain moisture, allowing the skin to function as an effective barrier against infection.

Some simple skin solutions can be made in your own kitchen from regular pantry items, meaning that you know exactly what you're putting on your skin and can tailor things for your skin type (see chapter eight for easy recipes!).

The unfortunate irony is that the more irritated and inflamed the skin gets the more likely the development of a sensitivity or even allergy to lotions, make-up, cleansers and so forth. Inflammation puts the immune system on high alert and that might mean that allergies develop that otherwise would not have been a problem. Managing both systemic and localised inflammation can significantly reduce symptoms of skin conditions including psoriasis, eczema, and acne.

Existing allergies and intolerances, both to externally used products and ingested foods, can increase systemic inflammation. Other triggers for inflammation and conditions associated with chronic inflammation include:

- Autoimmune disease
- Infection
- Environmental allergens
- Asthma
- Chronic peptic ulcer
- Tuberculosis
- Rheumatoid arthritis
- Chronic periodontitis
- Ulcerative colitis and Crohn's disease
- Chronic sinusitis
- Chronic active hepatitis.

Signs of Chronic Inflammation

Chronic inflammatory conditions affect how the body works at a cellular level, making metabolic processes less efficient, producing more toxic metabolites, and prompting abnormal growth of some cell and tissue types. Food allergies, itchy skin or hives, acne, and eczema can all be signs of systemic inflammation, as can high blood pressure, water retention, and headaches. Removing pro-inflammatory foods from your diet and favouring anti-inflammatory foods as part of a plant-based diet can help reduce inflammation and provide great sources of nourishment to facilitate healing and repair.

Inflammation and Acne

Preventing unhealthy inflammation can delay age-related tissue degeneration, meaning that your skin can stay healthier and look younger for longer. Controlling inflammation is also a great way to stop angry looking red pimples in their tracks.

These kinds of pimples are usually caused by a bacterial infection and are tender to the touch, swollen and painful. Some inflammation is normal in response to such an infection as immune system cells rush to the area to fight off the nasty microbes. In fact, whiteheads are caused by a build-up of pus, which is a combination of dead bacterial cells and white blood cells. Blackheads are created when there is an abnormal build-up of sebum and melanin.

In order to beat acne it is important to keep the skin clean and avoid touching pimples that appear infected as this can spread bacteria from one spot to another, giving rise to yet more infected and painful spots. Learning how to control inflammation also makes it easier to reduce your risk of chronic acne and acne scarring, and can help the body mount a more effective response to bacterial infection.

Acne Scarring and Inflammation

Inflammation increases the likelihood of acne scarring by altering the way that the skin heals. In the normal healing process a certain type of collagen is produced as a first defence to seal a wound and restore the barrier function of the skin. However, ongoing inflammation in the skin means that this more fibrous type of collagen continues to be produced, rather than the elastic, supple and healthy tissue that usually follows the initial wound closure.

While you don't want to stop all inflammatory processes happening, it can help to know how to steer your body towards lowering systemic inflammation and preventing persistent inflammation after an initial attack has been dealt with successfully.

A whole foods plant-based diet provides plenty of antioxidants and anti-inflammatory foods that help control inflammation. In addition, a whole food plant-based diet can help you avoid a vast array of pro-inflammatory foods, such as red meats, simple sugars, and dairy products.

Choosing a low GI diet free from dairy, meat, and other animal products can help decrease the likelihood of skin breakouts connected to inflammation, insulin resistance, and dairy allergy or intolerance. In one study, women with polycystic ovary syndrome who were given drugs to help improve insulin resistance also reported clearer skin (Ciotta et al., 2001).

Before looking at the best foods to eat to help fight inflammation, let's take a quick look at some key things to keep off your plates if you want to control those angry red zits.

Sugar - A Major Cause of Inflammation

A diet high in simple sugars prompts the body to produce large amounts of insulin in order to quickly move sugar from the bloodstream into cells. This influx of insulin is designed to help reduce dangerously high blood glucose levels, which is important because hyperglycaemia can damage blood vessels and other tissues, leading to strokes, heart disease and poor circulation that impairs wound healing.

Chronically elevated blood sugar also increases the formation of undesirable compounds called glycated proteins that can damage nerves, tissues in the eyes, and other parts of the body. This damage is why many people with poorly managed diabetes have deteriorating vision, blindness, nerve problems, and even erectile dysfunction, kidney disease, and immune system dysfunction.

Over time, chronically high levels of blood sugar cause insulin-producing pancreatic cells to become fatigued and less efficient, and even to die. A lack of insulin not only means that blood sugar levels are then poorly controlled but also prevents cells from taking up glucose, a vital fuel for the whole body.

Where both blood sugar and insulin are elevated, our cells can become resistant to the effects of insulin, making it harder for cells to actually take up the glucose needed to fuel normal metabolism. This results in chronic tiredness, muscle weakness, and cognitive deficits, as the brain relies almost entirely on glucose as its energy source.

Sugar's Not So Sweet for Acne Sufferers

How is excess dietary sugar linked to acne and inflammation? Well, when we eat a lot of sugar or simple carbohydrates, the body converts the excess into fat for storage in enlarged adipose cells. These fat cells produce pro-inflammatory chemicals such as interleukin-6 (IL-6) which create systemic inflammation that can exacerbate acne.

Dietary fat might make us fat but so can sugar, and both can cause an exaggerated response to trauma, infection, and injury that results in tissue damage, swelling, and an increased risk of acne scarring.

Sugar (particularly in the form of lactose in dairy products) can also feed undesirable bacteria in the gut, and lead to conditions such as Candida albicans (thrush) and increased inflammation which may trigger or exacerbate acne. See chapter 2 for more on the gut-acne connection.

While it's possible to eat a plant-based (vegan) diet that is high in sugar, it is a little less likely as many processed foods are simply not vegan-friendly and the majority of processed sugar is also not vegan-friendly as it is filtered through bone char. Less obvious sources of simple sugars can still be present in a plant-based diet however, in the form of white bread, pasta, potatoes, and even some supposed multigrain breads and products which are made using heavily milled flour that is quickly digested into simple carbohydrates.

Other Sources of Inflammation to Avoid

Sugar is not the only culprit behind increased inflammation. Certain fats (namely trans fats and some saturated fats), dairy, highly allergenic foods such as those containing gluten, and a number of meats and other animal-derived products can all increase inflammation.

This link between certain fatty foods and increased inflammation may due to the presence of toxins such as pesticides that tend to concentrate in animal fats, particularly in fish. It may also be a result of hormone residues in milk and meat products, and the disturbing effect of dairy products on gut flora (see chapter four).

Arachidonic Acid

As we've already seen how high glycaemic diets and insulin resistance can contribute to acne, it will come as no surprise that it makes sense to minimise intake of another possible trigger for insulin mismanagement, namely arachidonic acid.

Every time a cell is exposed to insulin its production of GLUT4 decreases (Flores-Riveros et al., 1993). GLUT4 is an insulin-regulated glucose receptor on the cell's membrane, which means that a depletion of this receptor makes cells less able to respond to insulin. Over time, insulin exposure can cause dramatic decreases in GLUT4, leading to the development of insulin resistance. Rather alarmingly, ordinary dietary exposure to arachidonic acid can cause a 90% suppression of GLUT4 (Tebbey et al., 1994).

Arachidonic acid is predominantly found in foods of animal origin and, while we can produce some ourselves (from linoleic acid), there is no clear dietary requirement for this fatty acid in humans. This suggests that if linoleic acid intake is sufficient, the removal of animal-derived foods may help some people avoid excess exposure to arachidonic acid and reduce acne symptoms.

Exercise

Next time you're tempted to eat a steak, run! No, seriously. Not only will you decrease your intake of arachidonic acid, exercise has also been shown to help increase the production of GLUT4 (sometimes by as much as 90%). This helps the body use insulin more effectively, thereby reducing a major trigger of acne (MacLean et al., 2002).

Exercise also helps increase circulatory health and the delivery of nutrients and oxygen to the skin. Staying active is also an important part of combating metabolic syndrome, and boosting mental health, which may itself be tied to acne and inflammation. One study found that aerobic exercise reduced a number of inflammatory markers, including IL-6, IL-18, and C-reactive protein (Kohut et al., 2006).

Acne, Inflammation and Mood

Stress and depression have both been linked to inflammation, which can exacerbate chronic health conditions and fuel a vicious cycle of feeling stressed about your health and gradually feeling worse physically (Lutgendorf et al., 1999). Those in stressful relationships or who are repeatedly exposed to negative professional experiences or social situations have been found to experience increased inflammation, while those who are well supported have fewer signs of inflammation in the blood (Chiang et al., 2012).

Inflammation and depression are potentially linked in the opposite direction too, with high levels of inflammation possibly triggering or worsening depression (Pasco et al., 2010; Gimeno et al., 2009). So, it seems that some of the things that cause or exacerbate acne may also be making you feel depressed, stressed, and anxious.

Practising guided meditation or undergoing cognitive behavioural therapy has been shown to help in chronic inflammatory conditions, particularly where inflammation is accompanied by stress, depression, and/or anxiety (Pace et al., 2009). Getting adequate rest is also important, as this downtime not only allows the skin to heal itself, it also reduces stress-induced inflammation (Meier-Ewert et al., 2004).

We've covered a lot in this chapter, including how inflammation arises in the body and why it matters, some key dietary, lifestyle, and environmental triggers for inflammation, and some suggestions as to what to do to reduce both localised and systemic inflammation. Check out the practical steps on the next page to get a reminder and summary of how to put this knowledge into action to help combat your acne and boost your general health and well-being.

Practical Steps

There are many things you can do to lower your levels of inflammation and reduce your risk of acne. Rather than feeling daunted by this list, pick just one or two and concentrate on having those things become habit before moving on to the rest.

You can start taking back control of inflammation by choosing to:

- Remove inflammatory triggers in your diet, such as alcohol and simple sugars
- Cut out animal based foods including red meat, dairy, and fish that may contain concentrated toxin residues, hormones, and allergens
- Reduce your intake of saturated and trans fats
- Eat a high fibre, low glycaemic index diet with plenty of healthy monounsaturated and polyunsaturated fats from nuts and seeds
- Use probiotics and prebiotics to correct intestinal dysbiosis tied to inflammation
- Consider using algal oil supplements to increase intake of anti-inflammatory DHA and EPA (long-chain omega-3 fatty acids)
- Try to reduce stress through mindfulness practice, yoga, exercise, a new hobby, or relaxation techniques including biofeedback
- Avoid using toiletries and cosmetics that contain irritants and allergens
- Stay hydrated and get enough sleep!

CHAPTER SEVEN: ANTI-ACNE & ANTI-INFLAMMATORY FOODS

In earlier chapters we looked at likely dietary triggers of acne and how drastic 'cleanses' may do more harm than good for our skin. Now we know what not to eat, it's time to focus on those foods that may actually help reduce acne incidence and severity.

A healthy, nourishing diet that contains adequate minerals, vitamins, fats, proteins, and other vital nutrients and beneficial phytonutrients can make a dramatic difference in terms of the frequency and severity of acne flare-ups and scarring. By providing the cells with antioxidants and hydration they are better able to carry out normal cellular processes and resist abnormal and undesirable cellular changes.

Nourished skin cells are also better positioned to maintain strong but flexible cell membranes that can more successfully defend the body from bacterial invasion. Infection of the skin's cells can cause angry red blotches, acne and more severe rosacea, psoriasis, and eczema.

Staying hydrated and maintaining overall health can have significant benefits for skin disorders including acne. Maintaining functional cell membranes plays a huge role in skin health, meaning that adequate antioxidant intake is essential.

Skin cells have a lipid membrane that contains both hydrophilic (fat-loving) vitamin E molecules and hydrophobic (water soluble) vitamin C. Together, these vitamins help protect the cells against oxidative damage, with vitamin C able to refresh the vitamin E molecules and maintain membrane stability after free-radical exposure.

Omega-3 is also important for maintaining healthy, flexible, and responsive cell membranes, as well as for numerous other bodily functions. As the body is unable to synthesise omega-3 or vitamins E and C, these nutrients need to come from the diet, as do numerous other vitamins and minerals needed for optimal skin health.

Diet and Skin Health

It's all well and good to recommend a healthy and balanced diet for skin health, until we start to scrutinise what balanced and healthy really mean. For the most part, this advice focuses on eating a diet rich in fruits, vegetables, and whole grains. Unfortunately, however, we can no longer safely assume that the produce on offer at the grocery store is as nutritious as it used to be.

Decades of over-farming, and the use of pesticides, herbicides and fungicides have all contributed to a situation where the soil in which our food crops are grown is often depleted of vitamins and minerals and contaminated with toxins. Research shows that levels of zinc, iron, copper, and magnesium have all decreased dramatically in wheat grain and soil in the UK since 1960 (Fan et al., 2008). Levels of other minerals, including nitrogen, manganese, and phosphorus are also influenced by the use of artificial fertilisers, affecting both the quality of food and dietary nutrient intake (Sheng et al., 2009; Watanabe et al., 2015).

Along with making sure that all produce is thoroughly washed before consumption, there are other ways to minimise exposure to toxins in food.

Organic Foods and Skin Health

Eating organic produce is a good way to optimise intake of vitamins and minerals and reduce the burden of toxicity on your body. Organic fruits, vegetables, nuts, seeds and grains only have themselves to rely on to thwart attacks from pests and, as such, build up higher concentrations of protective substances such as quercetin and other bioflavonoids. When we eat these organic foods we are also ingesting these protective compounds, instead of the pesticides found in non-organic produce.

Brightly coloured fruits and vegetables are a must for anyone looking to boost intake of nutrients that support skin health. This is because the colourful compounds that create beautiful blue, red, purple, and green plant foods also have exemplary antioxidant activity and a whole host of other health benefits. Even white vegetables and fruits can be a rich source of beta-carotene and other carotenoids, anthocyanidins, vitamins, and other protective compounds that help decrease inflammation and even facilitate better glucose metabolism.

Beta-carotene, vitamins C, E and A, along with selenium, zinc, lycopene and quercetin are all important factors in fighting off free-radical damage in the skin, slowing down the visible signs of ageing, and also helping reduce levels of histamine that can exacerbate acne flare-ups.

Choosing Fresh and Choosing Local

Although it is not always the case, choosing to eat local produce that has been freshly picked will usually mean less exposure to toxins and higher levels of nutrients. The reason for this is twofold: those producing these crops are less likely to have to use artificial means to grow things out of season; and the produce is not doused with chemicals to preserve it while the food is transported hundreds or even thousands of miles to reach consumers. Buying local also means that you are more likely to be able to talk to those who have grown the foods you are about to eat, allowing you to find out about their farming practices and encourage the use of vegan organic agriculture that works to enrich the soil over time.

Of course, not all organic standards are the same and so it is important to find out how legislation works in your area. Some producers of organic food may only be required to demonstrate a year of organic practice to have their soil certified, while others may still be able to use some herbicides on their property and retain organic status. Knowledge is power, so be an engaged consumer and advocate for your own health!

Dietary Fats and Acne

Another way to minimise exposure to toxins is to consider the food chain and toxic accumulation. Animals higher up in the food chain tend to concentrate toxins, particularly in fat stores, which is why some species of fish can have excessively high levels of mercury, lead, and cadmium. The provenance of animal products also makes a difference as fish from fish farms, or animals from feedlots are much more likely to be exposed to antibiotics as well as bacteria from unhygienic living conditions.

Fish and other seafood may also have been exposed to heavy metals from nearby garbage dumps and pollution in the ocean. As such, it is often simply easier to minimise toxin exposure by getting all the nutrients you need from non-animal sources (in addition to B12 supplementation, which is advisable even on an omnivorous diet).

This is not to say that plant-foods are immune to concerns about toxicity. Some plants grown on polluted soil can also accumulate toxins, oftentimes from agricultural run-off from nearby farms with livestock. The difference is that plant foods contain an abundance of nutrients that can help your body handle toxins more effectively, and most plant foods contain little fat, which is where toxins tend to accumulate.

Many people eagerly follow recommendations to increase consumption of oily fish, anticipating anti-inflammatory and anti-acne effects, only to find that this can makes acne worse. This may be a result of the concentration of toxins in many fish species and the resulting stress on the body, triggering oxidative damage, inflammation, and skin flare-ups.

Getting your fats from organic nuts, seeds, olive oil and coconut can be much healthier in terms of lowering the toxic burden and providing added nutritional benefits such as fibre, minerals, vitamins and phytonutrients that keep cell membranes happy and healthy.

Why We Need Healthy Fats

Cell membranes contain a variety of different fatty acids, and the make-up of these fatty acids strongly influences how well cell membranes function. The higher the concentration of unsaturated fatty acids the more flexible the cell membrane. A higher proportion of unsaturated fatty acids in cell membranes also improves the cells' response to insulin signalling as well as their capacity to control the transport of substances in and out of the cells.

Research suggests that certain essential fatty acids (EFAs), such as linoleic acid (omega-6), have an important role in maintaining the integrity of the epidermal layer of the skin. This is because these EFAs support cohesion in the stratum corneum and prevent water loss through the epidermis, helping to keep skin hydrated and structurally sound.

In the 1980s some researchers observed a tendency for acne sufferers to have lower levels of linoleic acid in their skin (Downing et al., 1986). This was thought to make these people more vulnerable to the development of acne lesions because depletion of this EFA in the skin is thought to be involved in follicular hyperkeratosis (Downing et al., 1986). This overproduction of keratin can result in blocked pores and acne. It has also been noted that high levels of sebum dilute linoleic acid concentrations, meaning that skin concentrations of linoleic acid may become insufficient even when dietary intake of the EFA appears to be adequate.

Low levels of linoleic acid also reduce the effectiveness of the epidermal barrier, making the skin more vulnerable to inflammatory substances (Cunliffe et al., 2004). As such, it may be helpful for acne sufferers to pay particular attention to foods in the diet that are rich in linoleic acid, while continuing to ensure an adequate intake of alpha-linolenic acid (omega-3). Sources of linoleic acid include:

Sesame seeds (toasted, shelled)	13.887g/67.25g
Pine nuts	11.349g/34.24g
Walnuts, English or Persian (dried)	11.302g/29.67g
Pumpkin and squash seeds (roasted)	11.259g/57.57g

In previous chapters we have also looked at the relationship between arachidonic acid (found in animal products) and acne development and outbreaks. By favouring plant-based sources of polyunsaturated and monounsaturated fats it is possible to limit intake of pro-inflammatory saturated animal fats and trans-fats and actively encourage skin health.

Fatty Acids, Blood Glucose and Inflammation

Eating a low-saturated-fat, high-fibre diet also appears to help with insulin sensitivity, according to a study published in the journal Diabetes Care (Oranta et al., 2013). The study examined data from 518 healthy individuals between the ages of 15 and 20 enrolled in the Special Turku Coronary Risk Factor Intervention Project (STRIP). Participants were enrolled in the study during infancy and received continuous education about dietary changes for heart health.

Researchers encouraged those enrolled to reduce their consumption of saturated fats and favour a diet higher in fruits, vegetables, and whole grains. The overall health and degree of insulin resistance was continually assessed, and those who had a higher intake of fibre and a lower intake of saturated fat showed better insulin sensitivity over the study, with benefits for heart health and acne.

By including plenty of fresh fruits and vegetables in their diet, these study participants were also ensuring good intake of antioxidants to help prevent lipid peroxidation and counteract metabolic diseases such as diabetes and cardiovascular disease.

Other ways to support blood sugar regulation and combat acne include making sure to consume enough protein, keeping to a low glycaemic index diet, and ensuring a good intake of EFAs from nuts and seeds. Algal oils are another great option for omega-3. Indeed, it is by eating algae that fish maintain such high levels of omega-3.

It's important to note that this recommendation is for a low glycaemic index diet, not for a low carbohydrate diet. A 2008 study involving male volunteers with acne found that the total lesion count reduced significantly in those eating a low glycaemic index diet compared to the control group; the same study also found a correlation between acne severity and dietary proportions of saturated to monounsaturated fatty acids (Smith et al., 2008).

Olive oil should also be a feature of any healthy diet as this natural oil is a rich source of mono-unsaturated fatty acids (MUFAs) and has been shown time and again to help reduce the risks of cardiovascular disease (CVD). This is in contrast to more easily damaged (oxidised) polyunsaturated fatty acid oils, and saturated fats, which may increase the risk of CVD. Olive oil also helps reduce fasting glucose levels, and fasting insulin levels, giving it a role in diabetes management and metabolic syndrome (Ryan et al., 2000).

By helping with blood glucose regulation, olive oil may have an indirect benefit for those whose acne is connected to poor blood sugar control. Olive oil has not been shown to directly contribute anti-inflammatory activity in the body however, and so it is wise to also include healthy polyunsaturated fats from sources such as algal oil, nuts, and flax and chia seeds for direct anti-inflammatory benefits.

Vitamins and Minerals for the Skin

Eating a healthy diet full of fresh fruits, nuts, vegetables and seeds provides an abundance of vitamins and minerals vital for skin health, but some nutrients do appear to be a little more important than others when trying to beat acne and other common skin conditions.

In some cases the emergence of a skin disorder can itself signify a deficiency in a particular vitamin. When such symptoms arise it is often the case that health problems are not just skin deep, demonstrating the premise outlined at the beginning of this book: your skin can be a sentinel for more systemic health issues.

Antioxidants for the Skin

Vitamin E

Vitamin E is one of the most powerful natural antioxidants. It can help quench free-radicals when taken internally and can help protect against free radical damage when used externally, assuming that skin lotions are formulated so as to actually penetrate the upper layers of the skin.

In particular, vitamin E is secreted through sebaceous glands as part of a clever mechanism that limits the harmful effects of peroxidated squalene. Squalene is a type of fat that is readily oxidised, causing an increase in skin inflammation linked to the development of acne lesions. Research suggests that acne sufferers have an unusually high ratio of squalene to other sebum constituents meaning that adequate vitamin E intake may be especially important for people with acne (Ottaviani et al., 2006; Zouboulis, 2001; Jeremy et al., 2003).

There is a significant correlation between squalene output and vitamin E secretion in the skin, and in areas where sebaceous glands are concentrated vitamin E secretion is continuous (Thiele et al., 1999). This suggests that our skin is actively using vitamin E as part of an antioxidant defensive strategy without us even knowing about it (Thiele et al., 2001).

Clearly, providing adequate amounts of vitamin E in the diet would appear to be beneficial not only for the maintenance of skin cell membranes but also for reducing the negative effects of squalene oxidation. This research may also help explain the positive effects on acne lesions seen with the use of topical vitamin E gels and creams.

Great natural sources of vitamin E include wheat germ (also a great source of zinc), almonds, hazelnuts, peanut butter, spinach, broccoli, kiwi, mango, and tomato.

Food, portion	mg/ptn	%DV
Wheat germ oil, 1 tablespoon	20.3	100
Sunflower seeds, dry roasted, 1 ounce	7.4	37

Almonds, dry roasted, 1 ounce	6.8	34
Sunflower oil, 1 tablespoon	5.6	28
Safflower oil, 1 tablespoon	4.6	25
Hazelnuts, dry roasted, 1 ounce	4.3	22
Peanut butter, 2 tablespoons	2.9	15
Peanuts, dry roasted, 1 ounce	2.2	11
Corn oil, 1 tablespoon	1.9	10
Spinach, boiled, ½ cup	1.9	10
Broccoli, chopped, boiled, ½ cup	1.2	6
Soybean oil, 1 tablespoon	1.1	6
Kiwifruit, 1 medium	1.1	6
Mango, sliced, ½ cup	0.7	4
Tomato, raw, 1 medium	0.7	4
Spinach, raw, 1 cup	0.6	3

*DV = Daily Value.
USDA, 2011.

Vitamin C

Alongside vitamin E, vitamin C is also a common ingredient in skin creams, with many manufacturers including this vitamin as a natural preservative. This means that vitamin C is typically not present in sufficient quantities to be considered medicinal. To protect skin health it is essential to ensure a good dietary intake, and this is best done by eating a variety of fresh fruits and vegetables. As with most vitamins, vitamin C is easily damaged by exposure to heat, light or air, making raw fruits and vegetables a great source of this nutrient.

Vitamin C is vital for the production of collagen and is used up rapidly by those who smoke or who are exposed to second-hand smoke. This is one of the reasons why smokers tend to get fine lines and wrinkles earlier than non-smokers. As vitamin C is also an antioxidant, smokers are more likely to incur free radical damage leading to earlier signs of ageing. Poor collagen production also affects the health of blood vessels, which can lead to impaired circulation to the skin. Decreased collagen synthesis adversely affects the skin's structural integrity and with it the skin's ability to stay hydrated, smooth and firm. Without adequate vitamin C, the skin can become cracked, increasing vulnerability to infection, inflammation, and acne.

Vitamin A (or pro-vitamin A, beta-carotene)

Vitamin A is another nutrient often found in skincare creams, sometimes in very high dosages as part of a prescription formula. In addition to being a potent antioxidant, vitamin A also helps maintain collagenous skin structures, and is not only popular with sufferers of acne but also with people looking to stave off visible signs of ageing.

In high doses vitamin A (retinol) may, however, cause the skin to become more susceptible to ultraviolet radiation (sun) damage. This means that it is wise to avoid sun exposure, or use a good sunblock, if using vitamin A topically or as a high dose medication.

Sources of pro-vitamin A tend to be present in high amounts in plant-based diets, with the body able to convert plant pigments called carotenoids into vitamin A as needed (El-Akawi et al., 2006). Beta-carotene and other carotenoids are antioxidants in their own right and are responsible for the vast array of colours of vegetables and fruits. Good sources of these protective carotenoids include dark leafy green vegetables such as kale and chard, and orange or purple foods including beetroot, peppers, and squash.

Importantly, vitamin A, like vitamin E, is fat-soluble, meaning that the body is only able to absorb vitamin A and pro-vitamin A alongside fat. As such, very low fat diets can have a range of negative consequences for skin health, partly due to a reduction in the absorption of beta-carotene and vitamin E. Even a little drizzle of olive oil on your salad will help with the absorption of these vitamins from peppers, kale, and other vegetables and fruits, as well as having benefits for insulin control.

Resveratrol

One fairly novel nutrient that has caused considerable excitement in recent years can be found in the skin of red grapes, as well as in blueberries, cranberries, and a few other plant foods. Resveratrol is an antioxidant that has gained plenty of attention for its possible role in helping lower the risk of cardiovascular disease as part of the Mediterranean diet. In recent years, resveratrol research has also revealed the potential for this compound to help treat acne, with one study noting that resveratrol reduced acne lesions by half!

Resveratrol's benefits for acne are thought to be due to its ability to reduce the growth of *Propionibacterium acnes* (a microbial cause of acne) and to decrease inflammation in the skin. One study involved patients with acne vulgaris using two types of facial gel on specific sides of the face for sixty days; one gel was a placebo and the other contained resveratrol. The patients and physicians didn't know which side was treated using which gel, but the results showed an average 53.75% reduction in their scores on the Global Acne Grading System (GAGS) on the resveratrol side, compared to a 6.1% reduction on the placebo side (Fabbrocini et al., 2011).

Resveratrol is a polyphenol that has been shown to significantly reduce levels of immunoglobulin factor-1 (IGF-1), and to aid insulin sensitivity (Fröjdö et al., 2008). It also appears to up-regulate (increase) transcription of the gene SIRT-1 (silent information regulator transcript 1), which can lead to a significant reduction in blood sugar independent of the activity of insulin (Sin et al., 2015). SIRT-1 also reduces inflammatory mediators such as C-reactive protein and interleukin-6 that may contribute to the angry red blemishes of some forms of acne.

In one study looking at patients with cardiovascular disease, those patients who took a resveratrol supplement for a year had significant reductions in inflammatory mediators and markers. These beneficial changes included a 26% decrease in levels of high-sensitivity C-reactive protein, a 19.8% decrease in tumor necrosis factor-alpha, a 24% decrease in the interleukin-6/interleukin-10 ratio, and a 19.8% increase in anti-inflammatory interleukin-10 (Tomé-Carneiro et al., 2012).

Laboratory tests have also revealed that resveratrol has a direct antioxidant effect and increases levels of glutathione and other antioxidant enzymes (Soeur et al., 2015).

Unfortunately, the benefits of resveratrol for the skin have only been seen in clinical trials using very high doses of resveratrol applied topically. To ingest that amount of resveratrol from wine you would have to drink about 250 bottles of wine a day, which would have some rather undesirable side effects, such as blood poisoning and death (Baur et al., 2006). Red grape juice also contains resveratrol, but the vast quantities of juice needed to reach clinical trial doses of the nutrient would contain a significant amount of sugar, making it counterproductive to health.

A resveratrol extract looks like the only good option to access benefits for internal health, and for acne the evidence currently only points to benefits from external resveratrol application.

While some laboratory studies have shown that resveratrol applied to skin cells (keratinocytes) helps protect against sun-induced cell damage, there is also evidence suggesting that resveratrol may actually increase the risk of ultraviolet light damage in skin cells (Pastore et al., 2013). This means that the use of resveratrol creams prior to sun exposure could be a bad idea. It may be that applying resveratrol topically as part of post-sun exposure skin care could help protect the skin though, with some research showing that this plant polyphenol can encourage the death of skin cancer cells (Potapovich et al., 2013).

See chapter eight for a red grape and potato face mask that could help soothe inflammation and protect against the bacterial infection that cause acne.

B Vitamins for Skin Health

The B vitamins are not only essential for the health of the adrenal glands, the nervous system, and digestion, they also play a major role in the health of the hair and skin. Many acne sufferers have been found to have low levels of folic acid and vitamin B12, possibly due to poor vitamin intake and/or poor absorption, and/or through an increased need for B vitamins due to hormonal and digestive issues and stress (Balta et al., 2013).

People with acne vulgaris who are prescribed isotretinoin appear to be at a higher risk of depleted levels of vitamin B12 and folic acid, with subsequent increases in homocysteine and the risk for cardiovascular disease (Gökalp et al., 2014). However, high doses of vitamin B12 have been linked to the development of acne lesions in some people, including in young children (Balta & Ozuguz, 2014). Ensuring a healthy, regular intake of vitamin B12 is essential, as deficiencies of this nutrient can lead to permanent nerve damage, anaemia, and other serious health issues. However, where acne suddenly develops or becomes worse following high doses of vitamin B12, it may be worth considering stopping supplementation to see if symptoms resolve, and then resuming supplementation with a lower, more regular dosage with careful monitoring of blood levels of the vitamin.

Biotin (B7) is another important nutrient for acne sufferers as it is a key component of skin, nails, and hair. Whether or not the presence of biotin in shampoos is beneficial remains unproven but as part of the diet it is vital for good skin health, as is niacin (B3), which is sometimes included in anti-ageing skin creams and creams for acne. Niacin appears to help decrease inflammation related to P. acnes overgrowth, with the potential to decrease symptoms of acne in some people

(Grange et al., 2009). However, where acne is associated with follicular hyperkeratosis, it is possible that niacin could either exacerbate or alleviate symptoms of acne as topical application of this vitamin can increase the production of keratin (Gehring, 2004). The wide-ranging effects of this single nutrient demonstrate the importance of understanding the cause of acne in order to apply appropriate treatment.

Pyridoxine (B6) can be particularly helpful to those whose skin tends to break out around the time of their period. This is because vitamin B6 plays an important role in balancing hormones, and extreme fluctuations in oestrogen/progesterone balance can be a trigger for acne. Vitamin B6 is often found alongside zinc in skin care supplements for women as premenstrual acne can sometimes indicate an excess of copper, a mineral antagonistic to zinc.

Minerals for Skin Health

Many macrominerals and trace minerals are vital for skin health, with zinc, selenium, and copper some of the most important as pertains to acne.

Zinc

Zinc is a required cofactor in hundreds of enzyme systems, including those involved in protein production, immune system activity, and healing. As such, optimal zinc levels can help reduce acne scarring and decrease vulnerability to overgrowth of P. acnes. Zinc is also thought to help regulate the activity of the sebaceous glands, making it useful in cases of acne caused by excess sebum. Hormone balance also depends on healthy levels of zinc, meaning that those whose acne is tied to elevated levels of androgens, premenstrual hormone fluctuations, stress, and menopause may find this mineral beneficial for skin health.

Among its many activities, zinc works alongside vitamin C in the synthesis of collagen, making these nutrients vital for strong, healthy, and supple skin. Plant-based diets are usually pretty high in vitamin C but, unfortunately, it can take a little while before the body becomes efficient at absorbing zinc from plant-based foods. This can mean that those adopting a plant-based diet would do well to pay extra attention to zinc intake in the first six months or so. Including a variety of nuts, seeds and legumes, as well as healthy whole grains, is a sensible approach to ensuring adequate intake of zinc (Amer et al., 1982).

Choosing plant-based sources of zinc has the added benefit of reducing potential exposure to heavy metals such as mercury, lead, and arsenic that are more likely to be present in animal-derived foods such as seafood. Aiming for at least one or two servings of nuts or seeds daily can help with zinc intake, alongside a diet rich in legumes and whole grains. It can also help to know a few superstar sources of zinc just in case:

Wheat germ	3.28mg/27g
Pine nuts	2.21mg/34g
Adzuki beans	3.1mg/170g cooked
Alfalfa sprouts	0.3mg/cup
Asparagus	0.57mg/half-cup cooked
Houmous	0.54mg/2tbsp
Lentils	2.51mg/cup cooked
Pumpkin seeds	4.4mg/60g roasted
Soybeans	4mg/80g roasted
Sesame seeds	3.32mg/30g toasted
Tofu	2.98mg/150g fried

Canadian Nutrient File, online search, Health Canada, www.hc-sc.gc.ca.

Carrying around roasted soybean snacks, sprinkling some wheat germ in your morning smoothie, and making a salad with sesame and pumpkin seeds, alfalfa sprouts, and a side of houmous offer easy ways to boost your zinc intake and help your skin.

Selenium

Selenium is another important mineral for skin health, functioning as an antioxidant that works well with vitamin E to mop up free radicals and prevent oxidative damage. These nutrients are particularly valuable for those with sun-associated skin damage.

The amount of selenium in foods can vary quite considerably as soil levels of the mineral are low in many countries, often due to depletion of the soil through poor agricultural practices. This means that, rather than having to do some serious investigative work to discover the origin of every piece of produce, it may be wise to have a daily dose of selenium in supplement form as an insurance against insufficiency. Some foods, such as Brazil nuts, are especially rich in selenium however, with just 6-8 of these a day providing the recommended daily intake of the mineral.

Copper

Despite its antagonistic relationship with zinc, we also need copper to maintain healthy skin. We only need small amounts of this copper, but this mineral is vital for the production of collagen as well as elastin, the protein that helps skin to remain elastic and flexible.

Anyone who takes a zinc supplement long term should be careful to also monitor copper intake. Most quality zinc supplements designed for long term use contain copper and zinc in a 1:7 ratio, i.e. 2 mg of copper to every 14 mg of zinc, in order to reduce the risk of copper deficiency.

Other important minerals for skin health include calcium, which helps with structural integrity in the skin, as well as with cell renewal and lipid barrier function. Chromium, magnesium, and biotin have been associated with a reduction in the risk of metabolic syndrome, which may help reduce inflammation and relieve acne symptoms (Barbagallo & Dominguez, 2007; Qiao et al., 2009; Geohas et al., 2007). Good sources of these nutrients include leafy greens, nuts, seeds, and pulses.

Anti-Inflammatory Foods

As we've seen throughout this book, there are many things that can trigger or exacerbate inflammation, be that in the body as a whole, or in the skin specifically. Fortunately, plant-based foods contain an abundance of anti-inflammatory compounds that can help counteract and prevent inflammation and contribute to the relief of acne.

Many phytochemicals display anti-inflammatory activity, including anthocyanins from blueberries and carotenoids from carrots. Indeed, anti-inflammatory compounds are found in a variety of kitchen staples, including:

Garlic	Fennel
Broccoli	Spinach
Onions (green and spring)	Yams / Sweet potatoes
Carrots	Collard greens

Cabbage	Bell peppers
Bok choy	Brussels sprouts
Cauliflower	Chard
Green beans	Kale
Leeks	Turnip greens
Olives	Blueberries
Strawberries	Mulberries
Cranberries	Raspberries
Acai	Cantaloupe
Grapefruit	Rhubarb
Pineapple	Papaya
Apples	Acerola cherries
Blackcurrants	Kiwis, kumquats, guavas
Lemons and limes	Oranges
Peaches	Avocados

Other anti-inflammatory foods include nuts, seeds, and legumes:

Cashews	Brazil nuts	Sunflower seeds
Flaxseed/linseed	Macadamias	Almonds
Walnuts	Hazelnuts	Chickpeas (garbanzos)
Lentils	Peas	Dried beans

Anti-Inflammatory Herbs and Spices

While fruits, vegetables, nuts, seeds, and legumes can all help combat inflammation, the real stars of the anti-inflammatory world are herbs and spices.

Turmeric is, perhaps, the best known of these, closely followed by ginger. Unfortunately, however, turmeric is very poorly absorbed and likely contributes little in the way of anti-inflammatory activity in typical dietary amounts. This has led researchers to investigate ways of enhancing the absorption of this spice so as to confer the benefits seen in laboratory studies. Specifically, it appears that reducing the particle size of turmeric and delivering it in an oil suspension can lead to significant increases in blood levels of curcumin, the main anti-inflammatory and antioxidant compound in turmeric (Shimatsu et al., 2012). Turmeric has also been shown to support liver function, with potential benefits for detoxification and relief from acne related to a build-up of toxins (Shimatsu et al., 2012).

Certain herbs and spices have long been associated with improved blood sugar regulation which, as we know, can have significant benefits for acne relief. It is only in recent years, however, that clinical research has been carried out to explore how it is that these herbs and spices exert heir beneficial effects.

Cinnamon is, perhaps, the best studied of these herbal therapies for diabetes and metabolic syndrome, with significant evidence to suggest its helpfulness in enhancing glucose metabolism. At 1-3g a day, cinnamon appears to help most diabetics improve blood glucose and lipid levels (Khan et al., 2003). Anyone using medication for blood sugar control should discuss the use of this spice with their physician as it may alter how much medication they need. Some forms of cinnamon may also be toxic in high amounts or when ingested regularly, particularly for young children.

Many herbs also have anti-inflammatory activity, including basil, oregano, rosemary, mint, and thyme. This means that you could mix up a wonderful anti-acne face mask comprising oats, kiwi, lemon and mint, or infuse olive oil, avocado oil, coconut oil, or almond oil with anti-inflammatory herbs for an extra-special balm to soothe inflamed skin. The added bonus is that you'll smell pretty delicious! Chapter eight in this book contains some simple recipes for anti-acne creams and cleansers using natural ingredients you likely already have at home. This chapter also looks in-depth at thyme's benefits for acne, and includes a recipe for a marigold and thyme anti-acne gel.

Grains and Skin Health

There are a number of factors to consider when choosing grains to support skin health. These include the potential for allergy, such as to wheat and/or gluten, as well as the glycaemic index of grains, their nutrient content, and their capacity to hinder the absorption of nutrients in other foods.

Some grains are more likely to offer benefits for those with systemic inflammation, despite not exerting anti-inflammatory effects themselves. This is because certain grains have a lower glycaemic index, meaning that they are less likely to trigger spikes in blood sugar and insulin and subsequent increases in systemic inflammation. Refined wheat flour products, including white pasta and bread, as well as some gluten-free foods made using refined rice flour can be very high on the glycaemic index and are best avoided by anyone with acne.

Better options include quinoa, steel cut oats, barley, buckwheat, rye, or brown rice instead of the processed versions which lack nutrients and cause blood sugar spikes.

A Prescription for Healthy Skin

The vast majority of people do not require daily vitamin and mineral supplements to support healthy skin. However, anyone with a health condition that affects nutrient absorption or the metabolism of certain nutrients should work with an experienced health care practitioner to ensure optimal intake of vitamins, minerals, and other nutrients such as fatty acids.

In some cases, adequate nutrition may be compromised by a lack of access to fresh whole foods, and this may make an insurance dose of minerals and vitamins an important part of staying healthy and reducing the risk or severity of acne symptoms.

For help figuring out optimal nutrient intake and how best to use natural health products to supplement the diet, it is best to talk to a qualified dermatologist with knowledge of the importance of vitamins and minerals for skin. Consulting a naturopathic doctor for help dealing with acne can also help identify nutrient shortfalls and devise a prescription for skin health, especially in cases where food sensitivities and/or allergies are suspected. In the meantime, a few simple changes in key areas can make a big difference to skin health and the frequency of acne attacks.

Ensuring adequate water intake and reducing or eliminating stimulants including caffeine, tea, and sugary caffeinated drinks is a good start to support skin health. Reducing your intake of simple sugars can also help, with the ideal being a diet that includes unrefined organic whole grains that have lower pesticide residues and are more nutrient-dense. On the next page you'll find more practical steps to help you eat to beat acne.

Practical Steps

We have covered a lot of ground in this book so far, and this gives you a lot of opportunities to make positive changes to support your skin. To get you started, here are a few key practical steps you can take right now to eat to beat acne:

- Ensure a good intake of plant-based proteins vs. pro-inflammatory animal proteins
- Work with a naturopathic doctor, nutritionist, or dermatologist to identify and address any shortfalls in vitamins and minerals essential for skin health
- Optimise fatty acid intake to reduce inflammation and boost cellular health
- Reduce your use of stimulants and alcohol
- Quit smoking
- Reduce your intake of sugar and refined carbohydrates
- Choose whole grains and low GI foods
- Stay hydrated!
- Eat the rainbow (i.e. include lots of brightly coloured foods in your diet)
- Incorporate anti-inflammatory herbs and spices into meals
- Eat seasonally and locally to increase nutrient availability.

CHAPTER EIGHT: SKIN SOLUTIONS FROM YOUR PANTRY

Lotions and potions can cost you an arm and a leg, so instead of splashing your cash on expensive miracle creams consider whipping up a few effective skin treatments in your very own kitchen. Once you get the hang of some basic principles you can quickly and easily make anti-acne face masks, skin toners, moisturising lotions, and a plethora of other great skincare products from things you have lying around in the fruit bowl, refrigerator and kitchen cupboard.

Homemade skin remedies are a great option for anyone with sensitive skin as you know exactly what is in your products, with no nasty synthetic chemicals or animal ingredients to cause skin irritation. And, even better, the only animal you'll be testing these on is yourself!

The following recipes don't require a lengthy and complicated search for ingredients but there are a few basic supplies you might want to have on hand to make things a little easier.

Basic supplies:

Mason jars or glass jars and bottles of different sizes
Small funnel
Blender
Cheese grater
Some hemp string or similar
Tea strainer
Cheesecloth/muslin (find it in your local health food store)
Soap dispensing pump

Voila! With these tools of the trade you can get to work making a range of great skin care products for yourself and for friends and family as unique, personalised gifts.

In this section we'll be looking at how to make:

- ❖ A simple salicylic acid clogged pore cleanser
- ❖ An antibacterial coconut and tea tree moisturising cream
- ❖ Potato and grape anti-acne face mask
- ❖ Oatmeal and grape anti-acne gentle body exfoliating scrub
- ❖ Super simple facial chemical peel
- ❖ Marigold and thyme anti-acne gel
- ❖ Oatmeal lavender bath bags
- ❖ Anti-inflammatory chai tea skin toner

Salicylic Acid Clogged Pore Cleanser

Salicylic acid is a common ingredient in many anti-acne creams. This beta-hydroxy acid encourages the removal of dead skin cells that can otherwise block pores and increase the likelihood of infection that leads to acne blemishes. By clearing away dead skin cells in a timely manner, salicylic acid may help prevent the skin's natural moisturiser, sebum, from getting stuck in the pores and causing inflammation and painful pimples.

As many of you will no doubt know, salicylic acid is the chemical used to produce aspirin, so you might think that you could just crush up an aspirin tablet and add it to your face cream. Alas, aspirin tablets contain a little more than just basic salicylic acid as first discovered in natural white willow bark.

For a good facial cleanser it is best to track down salicylic acid powder, which can be obtained inexpensively from most pharmacies or online. It is necessary to mix the powder with a little alcohol to make it dissolve. For some people a solution of salicylic acid is just too acidic and can cause irritation, so it is a good idea to add a natural pH balancer such as triethanolamine to achieve the acidity of solution that works for your skin. Do patch tests with different concentrations before using any solution on your whole face. Those with more sensitive skin will likely want to keep the concentration of salicylic acid below 5%. The recipe below works out to about 2% salicylic acid.

1/4 tsp salicylic acid powder
1/2 tsp alcohol
8 oz. cooled white tea (or green tea)

Mix the salicylic acid powder with the alcohol for about thirty seconds until it is dissolved, and then combine this solution with the cooled green tea. Store it in a glass bottle and use as needed.

For those using the pH balancer, two ounces of toner can be made using:

1/2 tsp salicylic acid powder
1 1/2 teaspoons of alcohol
11 tsps hot water or hot white tea
Triethanolamine (add two drops at a time until reaching pH 4)

To test the pH of your solution, pick up some litmus paper from your local pharmacy.

Clean your skin first and leave it slightly damp before applying your solution using organic cotton pads or a reusable soft face cloth. Salicylic acid needs to be left on the skin to work, so don't wash it off. After applying the salicylic acid solution, you can then apply your preferred moisturiser (if you have one) and the acid will get to work clearing those clogged pores.

Antibacterial Coconut and Tea Tree Moisturising Cream

Coconut oil is something of a godsend when it comes to natural skin and hair care. This oil is a fantastic moisturiser, can help soothe dry and itchy skin, is great for eczema, has antifungal properties, and can even be used as an emergency sunscreen as it has an SPF of about 8 (as does olive oil!). Solid at room temperature, coconut oil has a fairly high smoke point and is a good alternative to animal fats when cooking. It is pretty calorific though, and you still need your polyunsaturated fats for good health, so make sure to use coconut oil sparingly and to also include olive oil, hemp oil, and flax oil in your diet.

Anyone with oily skin and the pimples and acne this can cause may think it counterintuitive to use coconut oil as an anti-acne cream. However, coconut oil can be applied in the shower or straight after a shower to help nourish the natural skin barrier and manage moisture levels, actually reducing one of the triggers for excess sebum production. Add in a few drops of antibacterial tea tree essential oil and you've got a great acne cream for those areas of skin that frequently crack, blister and look angry and inflamed.

Tea tree oil can cause irritation when applied directly to the skin, drying it out and making infection and acne scarring more likely. Combining tea tree with the natural moisturising properties of coconut oil creates a fantastic antifungal, antibacterial, acne remedy that takes just a few minutes to make and is inexpensive and easy to use.

You will need:

1/2 cup coconut oil
20-30 drops of tea tree essential oil

You've got two options with this cream: use a powerful blender to whip up the ingredients (and be prepared to have your blender smell like tea tree for a while), or melt your coconut oil in a shallow Mason jar partly submerged in hot water and then mix in the tea tree oil while the oil is warm.

As it cools, the coconut oil mixture will solidify and you can simply scoop out a little at a time and work it into those problem areas. Avoid using it near your eyes as the essential oil could cause irritation.

Potato and Red Grape Anti-Acne Face Mask

Many of us know that a glass or two of red wine can help you forget about your acne, but that's not quite the intention with this red grape acne remedy. Instead, as we saw in the last chapter, red grape skins contain a powerful antioxidant nutrient called resveratrol that was found to reduce acne lesions by half in one study (Fabbrocini et al., 2011). The authors of that study have been careful to note that the resveratrol in wine is metabolised by the body before it reaches the skin, and there is only evidence of a positive effect on acne when resveratrol is applied topically.

This face mask is inspired by that research, in addition to evidence that resveratrol may be a useful skin treatment after (but not prior to) exposure to ultraviolet light. The amounts of resveratrol used in anti-acne studies are much more concentrated than you'll be able to mix up at home but, depending on your skin type, this red grape and potato mask could help calm down inflammation and tighten up the pores on your face. For those with skin that is dry and sensitive, try using the oatmeal base recipe instead.

1/2 cup red grapes (crushed, or well mashed)
1 small potato (finely shredded)

Substitution: use 1/4 cup unsweetened red grape juice.

After shredding the potato and crushing the grapes, mix these together in a sealable container and place in the refrigerator for about an hour to cool (or marinate the potato in the grape juice for about an hour). Take the mixture and carefully apply to your face, covering all the problem areas. Apply a cool, damp cloth over your face to reduce messiness, and let this sit for ten to fifteen minutes before gently removing the mask and wiping away any grape juice.

Applied morning and night, the acids in the raw potato and the resveratrol in the red grapes may help soothe acne, tighten pores, and even reduce the visibility of acne scarring.

Oatmeal and Grape Anti-Acne Facial

1/2 cup raw organic oats or oatmeal
1/2 cup crushed red grapes (or 1/4 cup red grape juice)

Ideal for those with dryer, more sensitive skin, this soothing oatmeal facial is almost as easy as making porridge. If using oats, grind these in a food processor before cooking them in a little water; use unsweetened rice, almond or hemp milk for added luxury. Let the oatmeal cool until just above room temperature then mix in the crushed grapes or juice and cover your face with the mixture.

Leave the mask on for fifteen minutes to help soothe areas of acne, dry skin, and/or sun damage and then rinse away with lukewarm water and a gentle cleanser or antibacterial soap.

The polysaccharides in the oats can help your skin to retain moisture and reduce dryness and sensitivity, while the resveratrol in the grapes can help reduce the spread of bacteria that cause acne and provide antioxidant protection to the skin.

Super Simple Chemical Peels for Acne

Acne scarring can lead many people to seek cosmetic dermatological treatments such as chemical peels even after their acne is resolved. These peels typically use alpha-hydroxy acids to strip away the top layers of the skin and encourage the body to regrow that skin with a smoother appearance.

Strong chemical peels can leave the skin inflamed and irritated and may even cause more scarring, meaning that it is important to only undergo such strong chemical peels under the guidance of an experienced dermatologist.

What many people don't realise is that the chemicals used in these treatments are typically derived from fruits such as pineapple and papaya. Lemons, limes, and oranges also contain these natural fruit acids that can help strip away dead skin cells and break down proteins to clear the skin and encourage the growth of healthy new tissue.

Pineapple and papaya are great options for home-made skin peels. This is because they also contain anti-inflammatory compounds including bromelain and papain which break down tough proteins, such as keratin, found in the skin. These fruit extracts may also help prevent redness and irritation by soothing the skin. If using these fruits, make sure to choose fresh fruit where the enzymes are still going to be active, rather than fruit canned in juice or syrup.

The easiest fruity chemical peel for acne is to apply a small amount of fresh lemon juice to areas of problem skin and then leave it to work for ten minutes before gently rinsing the area. The citric acid in the lemon acts as a gentle chemical peel.

You could also pulp fresh apple with added lime or lemon juice and use this as a mask on the face for five or ten minutes (or longer if desired). Other options for natural chemical peels include:

Fresh applesauce
Apple cider vinegar
Crushed blackberries
Tomato juice

Nature's pantry is also nature's beauty counter!

Marigold and Thyme Anti-Acne Gel

Looking for a scientifically validated effective acne relief treatment? Well, thanks to researchers at Leeds Metropolitan University in the UK, you might be in luck!

These scientists have discovered that thyme is a more potent antibacterial agent than plain alcohol, at least in laboratory tests on the bacteria that cause acne. What's more, thyme is anti-inflammatory, making it a great acne therapy for acne rosacea and adult acne which can leave the face looking red and swollen.

The scientists steeped thyme, marigold (calendula), and myrrh in alcohol to produce tinctures and then tested their effects on the bacteria that cause acne. After five minutes they compared the effects to those of plain alcohol and found that the most potent of the samples was that produced with thyme. The team then tested the thyme tincture for acne against benzoyl peroxide, the usual active ingredient in standard acne treatments, and found that thyme was, once again, more effective against the acne bacteria.

Acne treatments that use benzoyl peroxide can cause side-effects such as burning and skin irritation, but thyme has a gentler effect on the skin. While this may help you avoid undesirable side-effects and actually see more significant results, it should be stressed that no research has been done on the direct use of thyme on the skin, just on bacteria in a lab. This means that this natural thyme and marigold gel isn't itself scientifically validated, despite being based on some fairly strong evidence to support the use of these natural ingredients for skin health.

To make your own anti-acne thyme gel you will need

    8 sprigs of thyme
    8 marigold (calendula) flowers (optional)
    20 lavender flowerheads (optional)
    200 ml of water
    6 tbsps vodka
    15 drops tea tree oil (optional)
    1 sachet vegetable gelatine (or agar agar)

This recipe is a little more adventurous than those already outlined, and while it is recommended to include marigold and lavender for their soothing properties, and tea tree as an added antibacterial agent, these are optional, so you could just focus on the thyme.

To make this gel, set the water boiling, chop the marigold and lavender flowers and strip the thyme leaves from the stem (run your fingers down the stalk to gently strip the leaves). Add the flowers and leaves to a large bowl and carefully pour the hot water over the leaves and flowers, leaving the mixture to infuse for ten minutes, after which the water should have taken on the colour of the flowers.

Briefly mix the infusion in a blender and then strain it through cheesecloth into a fresh bowl. In a smaller bowl dissolve your vegetable gelatine or agar agar in a couple of tablespoons of cold water. Begin to slowly add the thyme and flower infusion to the gelatine or agar agar mixture, stirring it continuously to prevent lumps forming. When the mixture is smooth, add the vodka and tea tree oil to create a gel that can be poured, once totally cool, into a pump dispenser. If you have an old hand soap dispenser, perfect! Otherwise, you can buy a new pump dispenser or simply use a small glass jar and a mini spatula or spoon to scoop out the gel each time.

This thyme acne gel can be used twice daily to spot-treat acne, or more often if your skin is particularly inflamed. Stored in the refrigerator, this marigold and thyme acne remedy can last for up to six weeks.

Oatmeal Lavender Bath Bags

Acne doesn't just affect the face, of course, which is why it can help to take a soothing bath designed to offer relief from the itchiness and inflammation of back acne or acne on the buttocks, thighs and chest. One great way to calm down inflammation is to make bath tea bags using oatmeal and lavender.

All you need for this are a few squares of cheesecloth, a handful of oats and some lavender flowerheads. Place the oats and lavender in the center of each square of cheesecloth and then draw in the corners to create a little bundle that you can secure with string. Make sure the string is tightly wrapped and create a loop that you can hang around your bath tap. This way, as your bath is filling the water runs over the oats and lavender and all those good polysaccharides and essential oils will run into the bathwater. Alternatively, just drop the tea bag into the bath water and give it a good swirl.

Anti-Inflammatory Chai Tea Skin Toner

This is probably one of my favourite natural skin care recipes, largely because I drink a lot of tea and so almost always have some on hand. The beauty of this skin toner is that it lasts a long time if stored in the refrigerator. It also works as a great base for many other skin care products.

This acne remedy really is as simple as brewing up some unsweetened chai tea, which contains natural anti-inflammatory, antifungal, antiviral and antibacterial spices. After letting the tea steep for five or six minutes, strain the liquid into a glass jar to cool, and then store it in the refrigerator for later use.

To give this toner more of an antibacterial kick, trying adding in essential oils such as tea tree. For a soothing facial cleanser, try steeping some oats in the tea for a couple of hours before straining the liquid. To adapt this recipe for use as a great skin tonic for angry sunburn or other skin irritation or inflammation, puree some cucumber and aloe vera juice and mix with the cooled tea, then apply as needed.

And there you have it - simple natural skin care courtesy of your kitchen cupboards!

Great looking skin starts from within but these handy recipes can help soothe and cleanse and help your skin look and feel better while you get to work eating to beat acne with a plant-based diet.

References

Chapter 1: Getting to Know Your Skin.

Albano, R.E. (2004). Skin, Hair, and Nails: Structure and Function, CRC Press.

Balta, I., Ekiz, O., Ozuguz, P., Sen, B.B., Balta, S., Cakar, M., Demirkol, S. (2013). Nutritional anemia in reproductive age women with postadolescent acne. Cutan Ocul Toxicol, Sep;32(3):200-3.

Melnik, B. (2012). Dietary intervention in acne: Attenuation of increased mTORC1 signaling promoted by Western diet, Dermatoendocrinol, 4(1): 20–32.

Melnik, B.C., Schmitz, G., Zouboulis, C.C. (2009). Anti-acne agents attenuate FGFR2 signal transduction in acne. J Invest Dermatol, 129:1868–1877.

Chapter 2: How to Avoid Common Causes of Acne.

Barbagello, M., Dominguez, L.J., (2007). Magnesium metabolism in type 2 diabetes mellitus, metabolic syndrome and insulin resistance. Archives of Biochemistry and Biophysics, 458, 40-47.

Barnard, N.D., Scialli, A.R., Hurlock, D., Bertron, P. (2000). Diet and sex-hormone binding globulin, dysmenorrhea, and premenstrual symptoms. Obstet Gynecol, 95(2):245-50.

Bebakar, W.M., Honour, J.W., Foster, D., Liu, Y.L., Jacobs, H.S. (1990). Regulation of testicular function by insulin and transforming growth factor beta. Steroids 55, 6, 266-270

Brand Miller, J.C. (1994). The importance of glycemic index in diabetes. Am. J. Clin. Nutr., 59: ((Suppl)) 747S-752S.

Burris, J., Rietkerk, W., Woolf, K. (2014). Relationships of self-reported dietary factors and perceived acne severity in a cohort of New York young adults. J Acad Nutr Diet, Mar;114(3):384-92.

Crawford, M.A., Gale, M.M., Woodford, M.H., Casped, N.M., (1970). Comparative studies on fatty avid composition of wild and domestic meats. International Journal of Biochemistry 1, 3, 295-300.

Geohas, J., Daly, A., Juturu, V., Finch, M., Komorowski, J.R. (2007). Chromium picolinate and biotin combination reduces atherogenic index of plasma in patients with type 2 diabetes mellitus: A placebo-controlled, double-blinded, randomized clinical trial. American Journal of the Medical Sciences 333, 3, 145-153.

Hays, B. (2005). 'Female Hormones: The Dance of the Hormones, part 1.' in D Jones (ed.). The Textbook of Functional Medicine, Gig Harbour, WA: Institute for Functional Medicine.

Khan, A., Safdar, M., Ali Khan, M.M., Khattak, K.N., and Anderson, R.A., (2003). Cinnamon improves glucose and lipids of people with type 2 diabetes. Diabetes Care 26, 12, 3215-3218.

Low, Y-L., Dunning, A.M., Dowsett, M., Folkerd, E., Doody, D., Taylor, J., Bhaniani, A., Luben, R., Khaw, K.T., Wareham, N.J., Bingham, S.A. (2007). Phytoestrogen exposure is associated with circulating sex hormone levels in postmenopausal women and interact with ESR1 and NR1I2 gene variants. Cancer Epidemiology, Biomarkers and Prevention 16, 1009.

Pino, A.M., Vallardes, L.E., Palma, M.A., Mancilla, A.M., Yáñez, M., Albala, C. (2000). Dietary Isoflavones affect sex hormone-binding globulin levels in postmenopausal women. Journal of Clinical Endocrinology and Metabolism 85, 8, 2797-2800.

Ryan, M., McInerney, D., Owens, D., Collins, P., (2000). Diabetes and the Mediterranean diet: A beneficial effect of oleic acid on insulin sensitivity, adipocyte glucose transport, and endothelium-dependent vasoreactivity. Quarterly Journal of Medicine 93, 85-91.

Smith, R.N., Mann, N.J., Braue, A., Mäkeläinen, H., Varigos, G.A. (2007). A low-glycemic-load diet improves symptoms in acne vulgaris patients: a randomized controlled trial. Am J Clin Nutr, Jul;86(1):107-15.

Tham, D.M., Gardner, C.D., Haskell, W.I., (1998). Potential health benefits of dietary phytoestrogens: A review of the clinical, epidemiological, and mechanical evidence. Journal of Clinical Endocrinology and Metabolism 83, 7, 2223-2235.

Thiboutot, D.M., (1996). An overview of acne and its treatment. Cutis 57, 1 suppl., 8-12.

Qiao, W., Peng, A., Wang, Z., Wei, J., Zhou, A. (2009). Chromium improves glucose uptake and metabolism through upregulating the mRNA levels of IR, GLUT4, GS, and UCP3 in skeletal muscle cells. Biological Trace Element Research, 13 March.

Xie, J., Kvaskoff, M., Li, Y., Zhang, M., Qureshi, A. A., Missmer, S. A., Han, J. (2014). Severe teenage acne and risk of endometriosis. Hum Reprod, 29(11):2592-9.

Chapter 3: Is there any truth to these skin myths?

Addolorato, G., Mirijello, A., D'Angelo, C., Leggio, L., Ferrulli, A., Abenavoli, L., Vonghia, L., Cardone, S., Leso, V., Cossari, A., Capristo, E., Gasbarrini, G. (2008). State and trait anxiety and depression in patients affected by gastrointestinal diseases:

psychometric evaluation of 1641 patients referred to an internal medicine outpatient setting. Int J Clin Pract, 62:1063–9.

Barrimi, M., Aalouane, R., Aarab, C., Hafidi, H., Baybay, H., Soughi, M., Tachfouti, N., Nejjari, C., Mernissi, F.Z., Rammouz, I. (2013). Prolonged corticosteroid-therapy and anxiety-depressive disorders, longitudinal study over 12months, Encephale, 39(1):59-65.

Blatt, S.J., & Behrends, R.S. (1987). Internalization, separation, individuation, and the nature of therapeutic action. Int J Psychoanal, 68(pt 2):279-298.

Gray, P. (1990). The nature of therapeutic action in psychoanalysis. J Am Psychoanal Assoc, 38:1083-1097.

Gupta, M.A., & Gupta, A.K. (2002). Use of eye movement desensitization and reprocessing (EMDR) in the treatment of dermatologic disorders. J Cutan Med Surg, Sep-Oct;6(5):415-21.

Gupta, M.A., Gupta, A.K., Vujcic, B. (2014). Increased frequency of Attention Deficit Hyperactivity Disorder (ADHD) in acne versus dermatologic controls: analysis of an epidemiologic database from the US. J Dermatolog Treat, Apr;25(2):115-8.

Hughes, H., Brown, B.W., Lawlis, G.F., Fulton, J.E. (1983). Treatment of acne vulgaris by biofeedback relaxation and cognitive imagery. J Psychosom Res, 27:185–191.

Jung, G.W., Tse, J.E., Guiha, I., Rao, J. (2013). Prospective, randomized, open-label trial comparing the safety, efficacy, and tolerability of an acne treatment regimen with and without a probiotic supplement and minocycline in subjects with mild to moderate acne. J Cutan Med Surg, Mar-Apr;17(2):114-22.

Katzman, M., & Logan, A.C. (2007). Acne vulgaris: nutritional factors may be influencing psychological sequelae. Med Hypotheses, 69(5):1080-4.

Khan, M.Z., Naeem, A., Mufti, K.A. (2001). Prevalence of mental health problems in acne patients. J Ayub Med Coll Abbottabad, Oct-Dec;13(4):7-8.

Layton, A.M. (2001). Optimal management of acne to prevent scarring and psychological sequelae. Am J Clin Dermatol, 2(3):135-41.

Levy, L.L., & Emer, J.J. (2012). Emotional benefit of cosmetic camouflage in the treatment of facial skin conditions: personal experience and review. Clin Cosmet Investig Dermatol, 5:173-82.

Liebregts, T., Adam, B., Bredack, C., Röth, A., Heinzel, S., Lester, S., Downie-Doyle, S., Smith, E., Drew, P., Talley, N.J., Holtmann, G. (2007). Immune activation in patients with irritable bowel syndrome. Gastroenterology, 132:913–20.

Lombardo, L., Foti, M., Ruggia, O., Chiecchio, A. (2010). Increased incidence of small intestinal bacterial overgrowth during proton pump inhibitor therapy. Clin Gastroenterol Hepatol, Jun;8(6):504-8.

Loney, T., Standage, M., Lewis, S. (2008). Not just 'skin deep': psychosocial effects of dermatological-related social anxiety in a sample of acne patients. J Health Psychol, 13:47–54.

Magin, P., Adams, J., Heading, G., Pond, D., Smith, W. (2008). Experiences of appearance-related teasing and bullying in skin diseases and their psychological sequelae: results of a qualitative study. Scand J Caring Sci, Sep;22(3):430-6.

Mallon, E., Newton, J.N., Klassen, A. (1999). The quality of life in acne: a comparison with general medical conditions using generic questionnaires. Br J Dermatol, 140:672-676.

Pimentel, M., Hallegua, D., Chow, E.J., Wallace, D., Bonorris, G., Lin, H.C. (2000). Eradication of small intestinal bacterial overgrowth decreases symptoms in chronic fatigue syndrome: a double blind, randomized study. Gastroenterology, 118:A414.

Rubin, M.G., Kim, K., Logan, A.C. (2008). Acne vulgaris, mental health and omega-3 fatty acids: a report of cases. Lipids Health Dis, Oct 13;7:36.

Stokes, J.H., & Pillsbury, D.H. (1930). The effect on the skin of emotional and nervous states: theoretical and practical consideration of a gastrointestinal mechanism. Arch Dermatol Syphilol, 22:962–93.

Sulzberger, M.B., Zaidens, S.H. (1948). Psychogenic factors in dermatologic disorders. Med Clin North Am, 32:669-72.

Uhlenhake, E., Yentzer, B.A., Feldman, S.R. (2010). Acne vulgaris and depression: a retrospective examination. J Cosmet Dermatol, 9:59–63.

Viana, A.F., Maciel, I.S., Dornelles, F.N., Figueiredo, C.P., Siqueira, J.M., Campos, M.M., Calixto, J.B. (2010). Kinin B1 receptors mediate depression-like behavior response in stressed mice treated with systemic E. coli lipopolysaccharide. Neuroinflammation, 7:98.

Wang, Y., Kuo, S., Shu, M., Yu, J., Huang, S., Dai, A., Two, A., Gallo, R.L., Huang, C.M. (2014). Staphylococcus epidermidis in the human skin microbiome mediates fermentation to inhibit the growth of Propionibacterium acnes: implications of probiotics in acne vulgaris. Appl Microbiol Biotechnol, Jan;98(1):411-24.

Zhang, H., Liao, W., Chao, W., Chen, Q., Zeng, H., Wu, C., Wu, S., Ho, H.I. (2008). Risk factors for sebaceous gland diseases and their relationship to gastrointestinal dysfunction in Han adolescents. J Dermatol, Sep;35(9):555-61.

Chapter 4: Got milk? Got acne?

Adebamowo, C.A., Spiegelman, D., Danby, F.W., Frazier, A.L., Willett, W.C., Holmes, M.D. (2005). High school dietary dairy intake and teenage acne. J Am Acad Dermatol, Feb;52(2):207-14.

Bowe, W.P., Joshi, S.S., Shalita, A.R. (2010). Diet and acne. J Am Acad Dermatol, Jul;63(1):124-41.

Bowe, W.P., Logan, A.C. (2011). Acne vulgaris, probiotics and the gut-brain-skin axis – back to the future? Gut Pathog, Jan 31;3(1):1.

Broom, D.M. (2001). Effects of dairy cattle breeding and production methods on animal welfare. In Proc. 21 World Buiatrics Congress, 1–7 (Uruguay: World Association for Buiatrics).

Danby, F.W. (2009). Acne, dairy and cancer: The 5alpha-P link. Dermatoendocrinol, Jan;1(1):12-6.

Danby, F.W. (2010). Nutrition and acne. Clin Dermatol, Nov-Dec;28(6):598-604.

Darling, J.A., Laing, A.H., Harkness, R.A. (1974). A survey of the steroids in cows' milk. J Endocrinol, 62:191-7.

Hartmann, S., Steinhart, H. (1998). Natural Occurrence of Steroid Hormones in Food. Food Chem, 62:7-20.

Ismail, N.H., Manaf, Z.A., Azizan, N.Z. (2012). High glycemic load diet, milk and ice cream consumption are related to acne vulgaris in Malaysian young adults: a case control study. BMC Dermatol, 16;12:13.

Kern, F. Jr., & Struthers, J.E. Jr. (1966). Intestinal lactase deficiency and lactose intolerance in adults. JAMA, 195(11):927-30.

Newcomer, A.D., McGill, D.B., Thomas, P.J., Hofmann, A.F. (1978). Tolerance to lactose among lactase-deficient American Indians. Gastroenterology, Jan;74(1):44-6.

Schirru, E., Corona, V., Usai-Satta, P., Scarpa, M., Cucca, F., De Virgiliis, S., Rossino, R., Frau, F., Macis, M.D., Jores, R.D., Congia, M. (2007). Decline of lactase activity and c/t-13910 variant in Sardinian childhood. J Pediatr Gastroenterol Nutr, Oct;45(4):503-6.

USDA APHIS VS. (2007). Dairy 2007, Part I: Reference of Dairy Cattle Health and Management Practices in the United States, October 2007.

U.S. Department of Agriculture, Agricultural Research Service. (2011). USDA National Nutrient Database for Standard Reference, Release 24. Nutrient Data Laboratory Home Page: http://www.ars.usda.gov/ba/bhnrc/ndlexternal link icon; accessed 2/2/14.

USDA NASS, Data and Statistics: Quick Stats, www.nass.usda.gov/Quick_Stats/; accessed 3/21/13.

U.S. EPA, Ag 101: Dairy Production, www.epa.gov/oecaagct/ag101/printdairy.html, 9/10/09; accessed 2/25/11.

Vuorisalo, T., Arjamaa, O., Vasemägi, A., Taavitsainen, J.P., Tourunen, A., Saloniemi, I. (2012). High lactose tolerance in North Europeans: a result of migration, not in situ milk consumption. Perspect Biol Med, 55(2):163-74.

Chapter 5: Do cleanses really work for spot-prone skin?

Brzóska, M.M., Moniuszko-Jakoniuk, J. (2001). Interactions between cadmium and zinc in the organism. Food and Chemical Toxicology, 39:10; 967–980.

Nestle, M. (2007). What to Eat. North Point Press; 1st edition, April 17.

Valko, M., Rhodes, C.J., Moncol, J., Izakovic, M., Mazur, M. (2006). Free radicals, metals and antioxidants in oxidative stress-induced cancer. Chem Biol Interact, 160:1-40.

Chapter 6: Inflammation and Acne.

Chiang, J.J., Eisenberger, N.I., Seeman, T.E., Taylor, S.E. (2012). Negative and competitive social interactions are related to heightened proinflammatory cytokine activity. Proc Natl Acad Sci USA, 109:1878-82.

Ciotta, L., Calogero, A.E., Farina, M., De Leo, V., La Marca, A., Cianci, A. (2001). Clinical, endocrine and metabolic effects of acarbose, an alpha-glucosidase inhibitor in PCOS patients with increased insulin response and normal glucose tolerance. Hum Reprod, 16:2066-72.

Flores-Riveros, J.R., Kaestner, K.H., Thompson, K.S., Lane, M.D. (1993). Cyclic AMP-induced transcriptional repression of the insulin-responsive glucose transporter (GLUT4) gene: identification of a promoter region required for down-regulation of transcription. Biochem Biophys Res Commun, Aug 16;194(3):1148-54.

Gimeno, D., Kivimäki, M., Brunner, E.J., Elovainio, M., De Vogli, R., Steptoe, A., Kumari, M., Lowe, G.D.O., Rumley, A., Marmot, M.G., Ferrie, J.E. (2009).

Associations of C-reactive protein and interleukin-6 with cognitive symptoms of depression: 12-year follow-up of the Whitehall II study. Psychol Med, 39:413-23.

Hanninen, O., Kaartinen, K., Rauma, A.L., Törrönen, R., Häkkinen, A.S., Adlercreutz, H., Laakso, J. (2000). Antioxidants in vegan diet and rheumatic disorders. Toxicology, 155:45-53.

Kohut, M.L., McCann, D.A., Russell, D.W., Konopka, D.N., Cunnick, J.E., Franke, W.D., Castillo, M.C., Reighard, A.E., Vanderah, E. (2006). Aerobic exercise, but not flexibility/resistance exercise, reduces serum IL-18, CRP, and IL-6 independent of beta-blockers, BMI, and psychosocial factors in older adults. Brain Behav Immun, 20:201-9.

Lutgendorf, S.K., Garand, L., Buckwalter, K.C., Reimer, T.T., Hong, S.Y., Lubaroff, D.M. (1999). Life, stress, mood disturbance, and elevated interleukin-6 in healthy older women. J Gerontol A Biol Sci Med Sci,54:M434-9.

MacLean, P.S., Zheng, D., Jones, J.P., Olson, A.L., Dohm, G.L. (2002). Exercise-induced transcription of the muscle glucose transporter (GLUT 4) gene. Biochem Biophys Res Commun, Mar 29;292(2):409-14.

Meier-Ewert, H.K., Ridker, P.M., Rifai, N., Regan, M.M., Price, N.J., Dinges, D.F., Mullington, J.M.. (2004). Effect of sleep loss on C-reactive protein, an inflammatory marker of cardiovascular risk. J Am Coll Cardiol, 43:678-83.

Pace, T.W., Negi, L.T., Adame, D.D., Cole, S.P., Sivilli, T.I., Brown, T.D., Issa, M.J., Raison, C.L. (2009). Effect of compassion meditation on neuroendocrine, innate immune and behavioral responses to psychosocial stress. Psychoneuroendocrinology, 34:87-98.

Pasco, J.A., Nicholson, G.C., Williams, L.J., Jacka, F.N., Henry, M.J., Kotowicz, M.A., Schneider, H.G., Leonard, B.E., Berk, M. (2010). Association of high-sensitivity C-reactive protein with de novo major depression. Br J Psychiatry, 197:372-7.

Penwell, L.L., & Larkin, K.T. (2010). Social support and risk for cardiovascular disease and cancer: a qualitative review examining the role of inflammatory processes. Health Psychology Review, 4:42-55.

Ranjit, N., Diez-Roux, A.V., Shea, S., Cushman, M., Seeman, T., Jackson, S.A., Ni, H. (2007). Psychosocial factors and inflammation in the multi-ethnic study of atherosclerosis. Arch intern Med, 167:174-81.

Tebbey, P.W., McGowan, K.M., Stephens, J.M., Buttke, T.M., Pekala, P.H. (1994). Arachidonic acid down-regulates the insulin-dependent glucose transporter gene (GLUT4) in 3T3-L1 adipocytes by inhibiting transcription and enhancing mRNA turnover. J Biol Chem, Jan 7;269(1):639-44.

Chapter 7: Anti-Inflammatory Foods.

Amer, M., Bahgat, M.R., Tosson, Z., Abdel Mowla, M.Y., Amer, K. (1982). Serum zinc in acne vulgaris. Int J Dermatol, 21:481-4.

Arnaldez, F., Helman, L. (2012). Targeting the insulin growth factor receptor 1. Hematol Oncol Clin North Am, 26(3): 527–42, vii–viii.

Balta, I., Ekiz, O., Ozuguz, P., Sen, B.B., Balta, S., Cakar, M., Demirkol, S. (2013). Nutritional anemia in reproductive age women with postadolescent acne. Cutan Ocul Toxicol, Sep;32(3):200-3.

Balta, I., & Ozuguz, P. (2014). Vitamin B12-induced acneiform eruption. Cutan Ocul Toxicol, Jun;33(2):94-5.

Baur, J.A., Sinclair, D.A. (2006). Therapeutic potential of resveratrol: the in vivo evidence. Nat Rev Drug Discov, 5:493–506.

Chiba K, Yoshizawa K, Makino I, Kawakami, K., Onoue, M. (2001). Changes in the levels of glutathione after cellular and cutaneous damage induced by squalene monohydroperoxide. J Biochem Mol Toxicol, 15(3):150-8.

Cunliffe, W.J., Holland, D.B., Jeremy, A. (2004). Review Comedone formation: etiology, clinical presentation, and treatment. Clin Dermatol, Sep-Oct; 22(5):367-74.

Downing, D.T., Stewart, M.E., Wertz, P.W., Strauss, J.S. (1986). Essential fatty acids and acne. J Am Acad Dermatol, Feb;14(2 Pt 1):221-5.

El-Akawi, Z., Abdel-Latif, N., Abdul-Razzak, K. (2006). Does the plasma levels of vitamins A and E affect acne condition? Clin Exp Dermatol, 31:430-4.

Fabbrocini, G., Staibano, S., De Rosa, G., Battimiello, V., Fardella, N., Ilardi, G., La Rotonda, M.I., Longobardi, A., Mazzella, M., Siano, M., Pastore, F., De Vita, V., Vecchione, M.L., Ayala, F. (2011). Resveratrol-containing gel for the treatment of acne vulgaris: a single-blind, vehicle-controlled, pilot study. Am J Clin Dermatol, Apr 1;12(2):133-41.

Fan, M.S., Zhao, F.J., Fairweather-Tait, S.J., Poulton, P.R., Dunham, S.J., McGrath, S.P. (2008). Evidence of decreasing mineral density in wheat grain over the last 160 years. J Trace Elem Med Biol, 22(4):315-24.

Fröjdö, S., Durand, C., Pirola, L. (2008). Metabolic effects of resveratrol in mammals--a link between improved insulin action and aging. Curr Aging Sci, Dec;1(3):145-51.

Gehring, W. (2004). Nicotinic acid/niacinamide and the skin. J Cosmet Dermatol, Apr;3(2):88-93.

Gökalp, H., Bulur, I., Gürer, M.A. (2014). Decreased vitamin B 12 and folic acid concentrations in acne patients after isotretinoin therapy: A controlled study. Indian J Dermatol, 59:630.

Grange, P.A., Raingeaud, J., Calvez, V., Dupin, N. (2009). Nicotinamide inhibits Propionibacterium acnes-induced IL-8 production in keratinocytes through the NF-kappaB and MAPK pathways. J Dermatol Sci, Nov;56(2):106-12.

Gupta, O.P., Sing, S., Bani, S., Sharma, N., Malhotra, S., Gupta, B.D., Banerjee, S.K., Handa, S.S. (2000). Anti-inflammatory and anti-arthritic activities of silymarin acting through inhibition of 5-lipoxygenase. Phytomedicine, Mar;7(1):21-4.

Hong, J., Bose, M., Ju, J., Ryu, J.H., Chen, X., Sang, S., Lee, M.J., Yang, C.S. (2004). Modulation of arachidonic acid metabolism by curcumin and related beta-diketone derivatives: effects on cytosolic phospholipase A(2), cyclooxygenases and 5-lipoxygenase. Carcinogenesis, Sep;25(9):1671-9. Epub 2004 Apr 8.

Jeremy, A.H., Holland, D.B., Roberts, S.G., Thomson, K.F., Cunliffe, W.J. (2003). Inflammatory events are involved in acne lesion initiation. J Invest Dermatol, Jul; 121(1):20-7.

Khan, A., Safdar, M., Ali Khan, M.M., Khattak, K.N., and Anderson, R.A., (2003). Cinnamon improves glucose and lipids of people with type 2 diabetes. Diabetes Care 26, 12, 3215-3218.

McCarty, M. (1999). Vegan proteins may reduce risk of cancer, obesity, and cardiovascular disease by promoting increased glucagon activity. Med. Hypotheses, 53(6): 459–85.

Oranta, O., Pahkala, K., Ruottinen, S., Niinikoski, H., Lagström, H., Viikari, J.S., Jula, A., Loo, B.M., Simell, O., Rönnemaa, T., Raitakari, O.T. (2013). Infancy-onset dietary counseling of low-saturated-fat diet improves insulin sensitivity in healthy adolescents 15-20 years of age: the Special Turku Coronary Risk Factor Intervention Project (STRIP) study. Diabetes Care, 36:2952-2959.

Ottaviani, M., Alestas, T., Flori, E., Mastrofrancesco, A., Zouboulis, C.C., Picardo, M. (2006). Peroxidated squalene induces the production of inflammatory mediators in HaCaT keratinocytes: a possible role in acne vulgaris. J Invest Dermatol, Nov; 126(11):2430-7.

Pastore, S., Lulli, D., Maurelli, R., Dellambra, E., De Luca, C., Korkina, L.G. (2013). Resveratrol induces long-lasting IL-8 expression and peculiar EGFR activation/distribution in human keratinocytes: mechanisms and implications for skin administration. PLoS One, 8(3):e59632.

Potapovich, A.I., Kostyuk, V.A., Kostyuk, T.V., de Luca, C., Korkina, L.G. (2013). Effects of pre- and post-treatment with plant polyphenols on human keratinocyte responses to solar UV. Inflamm Res, Aug;62(8):773-80.

Schneider, I., & Bucar, F. (2005). Lipoxygenase inhibitors from natural plant sources. Part 1: Medicinal plants with inhibitory activity on arachidonate 5-lipoxygenase and 5-lipoxygenase[sol]cyclooxygenase. Phytother Res, Feb;19(2):81-102.

Sheng, J.P., Liu, C., Shen, L. (2009). Analysis of some nutrients and minerals in organic and traditional cherry tomato by ICP-OES method. Guang Pu Xue Yu Guang Pu Fen Xi, Aug;29(8):2244-6.

Shimatsu, A., Kakeya, H., Imaizumi, A., Morimoto, T., Kanai, M., Maeda, S. (2012). Clinical application of "curcumin", a multi-functional substance. Anti-Aging Med, 9(2), 75-83.

Sin, T.K., Yung, B.Y., Siu, P.M. (2015). Modulation of SIRT1-Foxo1 Signaling axis by Resveratrol: Implications in Skeletal Muscle Aging and Insulin Resistance. Cell Physiol Biochem, 35(2):541-52.

Smith, R.N., Braue, A., Varigos, G.A., Mann, N.J. (2008). The effect of low glycemic load diet on acne vulgaris and the fatty acid composition of skin surface triglycerides. J Dermatol Sci, 50:41–52.

Soeur, J., Eilstein, J., Léreaux, G., Jones, C., Marrot, L. (2015). Skin resistance to oxidative stress induced by resveratrol: From Nrf2 activation to GSH biosynthesis. Free Radic Biol Med, Jan;78:213-23.

Thiele, J.J, Weber, S.U., Packer, L. (1999). Sebaceous gland secretion is a major physiologic route of vitamin E delivery to skin. J Invest Dermatol, Dec;113(6):1006-10.

Thiele, J.J., Schroeter, C., Hsieh, S.N., Podda, M., Packer, L. (2001). The antioxidant network of the stratum corneum. Curr Probl Dermatol, 29:26-42.

Tomé-Carneiro, J., Gonzálvez, M., Larrosa, M., Yáñez-Gascón, M.J., García-Almagro, F.J., Ruiz-Ros, J.A., García-Conesa, M.T., Tomás-Barberán, F.A., Espín, J.C. (2012). One-year consumption of a grape nutraceutical containing resveratrol improves the inflammatory and fibrinolytic status of patients in primary prevention of cardiovascular disease. Am J Cardiol, Aug 1;110(3):356-63.

Watanabe, M., Ohta, Y., Licang, S., Motoyama, N., Kikuchi, J. (2015). Profiling contents of water-soluble metabolites and mineral nutrients to evaluate the effects of pesticides and organic and chemical fertilizers on tomato fruit quality. Food Chem, Feb 15;169:387-95.

Zouboulis, C.C. (2001). Is acne vulgaris a genuine inflammatory disease? Dermatology, 203(4):277-9.

Zouboulis, C.C., Nestoris, S., Adler, Y.D., et al. (2003). A new concept for acne therapy: a pilot study with zileuton, an oral 5-lipoxygenase inhibitor. Arch Dermatol, May; 139(5):668-70.

Chapter 8: More skin-solutions - from your pantry!

Fabbrocini, G., Staibano, S., De Rosa, G., Battimiello, V., Fardella, N., Ilardi, G., La Rotonda, M.I., Longobardi, A., Mazzella, M., Siano, M., Pastore, F., De Vita, V., Vecchione, M.L., Ayala, F. (2011). Resveratrol-containing gel for the treatment of acne vulgaris: a single-blind, vehicle-controlled, pilot study. Am J Clin Dermatol, Apr 1;12(2):133-41.

Leeds Metropolitan University. Thyme for a more natural cure to acne, 27 March 2012. Accessed online June 12th 2014: http://www.leedsmet.ac.uk/news/thyme-for-a-more-natural-cure-to-acne27032012.htm.

ABOUT THE AUTHOR

As a teenager, I was beleaguered with acne-riddled skin which, on top of my propensity for flushing bright red at the drop of a hat, meant that I was extremely self-conscious. I tried all manner of noxious chemical 'solutions' but the more facial scrubs, washes, ointments, and masks I put on my skin the worse it seemed to get. The irony was that the more of my meagre money I spent on these acne treatments the more stressed I became and the more breakouts I had.

The solution? I stopped stressing about it, quit using make-up to cover up my blotchy skin, and no longer spent money on things that promised the world and did nothing for me. In short, I focused on other things, arguably more important things and, guess what? My skin improved.

Now, OK, you may just think that the closing of my teenage years meant that hormones settled and my skin became clearer naturally but my story is all too familiar for those in their mid-twenties, mid-thirties, and even their forties as they give up a lifelong fixation on having perfect skin and find that shifting their focus is the best remedy they've ever tried.

Of course, I'm not simply advocating giving up on having healthy skin, I'm just saying that there may be a better way that is free, has instant benefits, and has desirable side-effects rather than troublesome complications associated with some acne medications.

The secret? It's not a secret. Eat well, sleep well, use natural and gentle products, relax, breathe and live with kindness and your skin will reflect that state of inner calm.

"But my life's so stressful! How do I find time to relax and eat well and and and...?"

Don't fret; I made my changes during my finals in my first degree! Whatever your daily stresses, take things slowly, treat yourself with kindness, and you'll get there, or not, and that's OK too.

The reason I wrote this book is so that, for less than the price of the latest miracle acne cream, I could help you find some simple solutions and put you on the path to great looking skin!

Disclaimer

The information provided in this book is designed to support, not replace, the relationship that exists between a patient and their health professional. This information is solely for informational and educational purposes. The publication of this information does not constitute the practice of medicine, and this information does not replace the advice of your physician or other health care provider. Neither the author nor publisher(s) of this book take responsibility for any possible consequences from any treatment, procedure, exercise, dietary modification, action or application of medication which results from reading this site. Always speak with your primary health care provider before engaging in any form of self-treatment.

To stay up to date with the science on diet and dermatology visit www.naturallyhealthyskin.org.

Made in the USA
Coppell, TX
28 October 2024

39271066R10063